Dynamic Menopause

Also by Beth MacEoin and published by Help Yourself

Come Alive: Your Six Point Plan for
Lasting Health and Energy

Dynamic Menopause

Beth MacEoin

Hodder & Stoughton
LONDON SYDNEY AUCKLAND

British Library Cataloguing in Publication Data
A record for this book is available from the British Library

ISBN 0 340 75687 X

Typeset by Avon Dataset Ltd, Bidford-on-Avon, Warks

Printed and bound in Great Britain by
The Guernsey Press Co. Ltd, Channel Isles

Hodder & Stoughton
A Division of Hodder Headline Ltd
338 Euston Road
London NW1 3BH

To the memory of my mother Nancy

Contents

Acknowledgments   xi
Introduction   1

1 Menopause: Threat or Opportunity?   5
Rolling back the years: outmoded perspectives on menopause   8
Sexual healing: early days of HRT   10
Seizing fresh opportunities: the alternative viewpoint   12
The importance of balance   14
A fresh perspective on the value of symptoms   16

2 Understanding Menopause   18
Positive perspectives on menopause   19
All you wanted to know about menopause and were   20
   afraid to ask!
Puberty as a mirror image of menopause   24
Positive aspects of menopause   29
Moving with the flow   31
Taking action   31

3 Mind over Matter: Preparation for Menopause   34
  Forever young or forever healthy?   35
  You are as old as you feel   37
  The impact of stress on health and vitality   41
  The nature of stress   42
  Stress-busting techniques   44
  Evaluating stress   45
  Simple techniques for coping with personal stress   46
  Simple techniques for coping with work-related stress   49
  General stress-proofing techniques: the relaxation response   54
  Relaxation techniques   57

4 Eating for the Long Run   62
  Why what we eat is of central importance as we move   63
    through menopause
  The basic foundation of sound nutrition at menopause   65
  Eating for healthy bones   79
  Eating for a healthy heart   82
  To supplement or not to supplement?   86
  Anti-ageing nutrients at a glance   88

5 Moving On Up: the Basic Benefits of Exercise   92
  Body maintenance   93
  Freedom from boundaries   95
  Fringe benefits of body conditioning at menopause   96
  Exercise and bone density   98
  Exercise and heart health   100
  Exercise and emotional well-being   102
  Getting moving: basic issues   103
  Whole-body approaches to exercise   108

6 The Medicated Menopause: the Pros and Cons of   115
    Hormone Replacement Therapy
  Menopause from a conventional medical perspective   116
  The conventional view and treatment of osteoporosis   118
  The basic background to osteoporosis   118

Heart health and HRT 121
Using hormone replacement therapy 123
Menopause from an alternative medical perspective 125
The natural progesterone debate 126
A question of balance: the nature of oestrogen dominance 128
Alternative routes of support: herbal and homoeopathic 130
medicines
Effective strategies for deciding on an appropriate course 132
of treatment for menopausal problems
The broader picture: deeper questions relating to the use 134
of HRT

7 Alternative Self-Help for Short-Term Symptoms 137
Hot flushes 138
Night sweats 142
Anxiety and panic attacks 144
Sleep disturbance 152
Fatigue 156
Fluid retention 165
Loss of libido 168
Mood swings and depression 173

Recommended Reading 184
Useful Addresses 186
Index 191

Acknowledgments

My warmest thanks are due to the following, without whose help this book would have been a less pleasurable experience to write. The publishing team at Hodder and Stoughton have been a continuing delight to work alongside, with special thanks being due to Judith Longman and Rebecca Russel Ponte for their warmth, sensitivity and professionalism. As always, special thanks are due to my agent, Teresa Chris, who has been an enduring source of encouragement, enthusiasm and inspiration over the course of many books. In addition, special mention should be made of Dr Anand and Dr Anthea Anand, both of whom have given so generously of their time and professional expertise in looking over specific chapters of this manuscript. Last, but never least, all my love and thanks to my husband, Denis, who has shown himself to be the true hero that he is over the course of this year. Without his constant advice, encouragement, and moral and practical support I doubt whether a single word of any of my books would have become a reality.

Introduction

How would you feel if you were told that you could be fitter, stronger, and generally healthier at menopause than at any other time in your life? Although this may sound a tall order, and may directly challenge some unwelcome negative assumptions we may have had lurking at the backs of our minds, there is growing evidence to suggest that a dynamic menopause is possible. The secret is to have enough appropriate information at our fingertips, and the resolve to act on it in preparation for this vitally important mid-life transition. When we do this, we can be astonished to discover that this significant watershed can be one of the most extraordinary turning points in our lives.

Writing this book has been inspired by my own very personal discovery of how we can be extremely mistaken in thinking of health as being the exclusive possession of the young, as the traditional belief has it. In the past there has been a marked tendency to think of zest, vitality, and sexual allure and confidence as belonging to those who are still under the age of thirty, with middle age being synonymous with a more passive and less zestful approach to life.

In my own experience this could not be further from the truth, and I am keenly aware as I treat large numbers of patients that I am not alone.

I grew up as a totally unfit, overweight, painfully shy child, who not surprisingly turned into an even more unhealthy, unconfident young adult. Constantly suffering from one minor ailment after another, while dealing with the challenges of an early marriage, working full-time, and setting up a home, I limped through my twenties aware that something was severely limiting my life and hampering my potential, but didn't have a clue to know where to start in order to make the necessary changes.

The crucial turning point came in my thirties when I began to train as a homoeopath, and started consciously to eat well and get physically fit for the first time in my life. This proved to be a cumulative process, and as the years have gone by a positive transformation has taken place that would have seemed impossible to me in my teens. Now I am closer to fifty than to forty, I am stronger, fitter and more at ease with my body than at any other phase of my life. This doesn't mean to say that there aren't problems that have to be dealt with, or that life has become a breeze, since mid-life presents personal challenges that can sometimes feel overwhelming. However, if we know the steps we need to take in order to support ourselves in meeting these challenges, the benefits are enormous, and we are free to move on with our lives having gained greater strength and confidence.

This might be all very well and good, but we might ask, what has this really got to do with a discussion of menopause? The answer is a very great deal, since I am now extremely aware that the problems I was grappling in my twenties were the very same issues that surface with a vengeance for women who are approaching and experiencing menopause. These are connected to questions about identity, self-image, ability to welcome change, and possibilities for satisfying self-expression, as well as a profound need to understand what practical steps we can take to support and strengthen our bodies. While we need solid information to help us deal with any symptoms that may commonly arise in relation to menopause, we also need to consider what these physical sensations could be telling us about as yet unresolved issues.

Menopause provides us with a startling opportunity for change,

2

a time when we can explore issues from our past that may have been hampering us in moving forward, and a crossroads at which we can focus on the shape we want our future to take. Rather than letting things drift into a hazy future, relying on hormone replacement therapy (HRT) to temporarily suppress symptoms, and vaguely hoping all will be well, why not use this as a vital opportunity to take the necessary steps that will carry us forward into the next phase of our lives?

This book has been designed to provide a basic guide to the information that we need in order to make these crucial choices. In it you will find the mixed approach that is needed to cover some of the most important issues that arise in connection with menopause.

What follows is not a list of common menopausal problems with possible solutions; it is much more of a general approach offering a broad perspective on the most appropriate tools needed to support us through this transitional phase safely to the other side. Practical information is given where needed about the arguments for and against the use of HRT, natural progesterone cream, and alternative therapies, as well as basic nutritional steps that need to be taken on board if we want to give our bodies maximum support and resilience. In addition, there is a discussion of the importance of physical fitness, with a run down of possible options available to us if this is the first time we are considering becoming more physically active.

Practical merits of an alternative medical approach are explored, paying particular attention to how this is especially relevant to helping us resolve psychological as well as physical issues that commonly arise in connection with menopause.

Perhaps most importantly of all, this book has been written in order to focus on some of the issues that may not previously have been sufficiently brought into the open. These are basically connected to the view that menopause should be presented, not as something that needs to be fought and denied for as long as possible (an approach that can be associated with conventional medical attitudes), but as giving us a focus for making positive changes in our lives.

After all, since women are living longer, we can expect to experience a substantial proportion of our lives in our post-menopausal years. Why not concentrate on ways of making this phase of life one of the most rewarding and satisfying we are likely to experience?

1

Menopause:
Threat or Opportunity?

Four years ago a very close friend said something to me that I have never forgotten, and I firmly believe it has a very special relevance to any woman who is contemplating menopause. The statement itself was very simple and direct: that the word 'change' when written in Chinese can be read one of two opposing ways. When interpreted in one way the word can be translated to mean 'threat'; read another way it will spell 'opportunity'. The simplicity and profound meaning of this statement was quite overwhelming to me, since I am extremely aware that the way in which we respond to change can determine the eventual outcome of that experience to an extraordinary degree. This is also likely to be even more true of any change that we perceive as being thrust upon us, rather than those we initiate for ourselves.

During an initial appointment with a patient I will often ask them what they fear most. Without a doubt, I would say the most common focus of dread and terror for most people is one of feeling out of control, or not being able to do anything to change their situation. If we think of menopause from this perspective and regard it as life-changing event which we are powerless to opt out of, and feel that it is initiating changes in our bodies, minds and emotions that make us feel we are spinning out of control, of course we are likely to feel extremely fearful, uneasy and threatened.

This unwelcome feeling is likely to be doubled in intensity if we also associate menopause with feelings of sadness and grief over the loss of our youth. If we approach menopause from this perspective, it is almost certainly going to involve a difficult transition because of all of the negative associations that are being projected on to it.

Fortunately for us, the reverse is also true. In other words, embracing the change that menopause presents us with as an opportunity for re-evaluation and renewal can radically alter the sort of experience that follows. This may sound all very well and good, but in order to make this a reality, we need practical, realistic and workable advice on how to make this attractive idea into a reality.

This is where *Dynamic Menopause* hopefully plays an important role, since I sincerely hope it informs each reader about the realistic choices that are available to them. After all, we can only feel genuinely empowered in making an important decision when we are making an informed choice. This is a very different situation to following one avenue of advice when we are unaware of what alternative routes of action are available to us that might be even more beneficial.

Even more importantly, while *Dynamic Menopause* has been written from a deliberately responsible perspective, giving the necessary weight and attention to discussions about serious health considerations such as heart disease and osteoporosis, it also spends a significant amount of time considering broader issues that are sometimes overlooked by the conventional medical approach. In other words, the information to be found in this book has been shaped from a genuinely holistic perspective, paying attention to the ways in which our minds, bodies and emotions are intimately interlinked.

The positive result is that all of the suggestions presented are made with the aim of restoring the whole system to a state of health, rather than treating one problem at the expense of creating another. This is as true of the sections on nutrition and exercise as it is of alternative medical options, since the emphasis is deliberately placed on including measures that will work as efficiently and effectively as possible, while not forgetting that they also need to be gentle and without any obvious side effects.

Attention is also paid to the importance of taking suitable preventive action where appropriate. This is done from a conviction that the most positive way of feeling we are taking control of a situation is surely to anticipate potential difficulties at an early stage. If we take this course of action they can be dealt with more decisively and swiftly than they would if they were allowed to develop into more full-blown problems.

The very fact of taking an active stance in confronting issues is likely to play an important role in making us feel empowered and more positive about the impact we can have in shaping our experience of health and vitality. After all, fear is often bound up with feeling powerless to influence whatever situation we perceive ourselves to be in. What is worse, this sense of passivity can also lead to depression as we begin to turn our frustration and resentment inwards, which inevitably undermines our levels of confidence and self-esteem.

However, if we begin to see menopause as a crucial opportunity for change where we have a range of choices available to us, this can immediately give us a sense of purpose and optimism. After all, one of the genuine advantages of being in mid-life is that we have a wealth of experience behind us that we can benefit from. We will have had more than half a lifetime of making life choices already, and probably the wisdom of more than a few mistakes and less than positive choices as well to learn from. By the time we hit menopause there will still be a host of new challenges to be met, but this situation is in sharp contrast to the equivalent emotional and physical turmoil of puberty.

When we face puberty we have to go through all of the confusion, mood swings, and seeking for self-knowledge and identity without the benefit of any extended context of experience against which we can balance any of our choices. There is also the inevitable tendency at puberty to refuse to listen to advice that is being offered, however well-meaning that advice is intended to be. The compensation, of course, is that when we are in our teens there is the unspoken assumption that we have years ahead within which we can find our way, and so we can afford to take our time to find ourselves.

On the other hand, by the time we are approaching menopause, we need to be focused in making our choices so that we have the maximum chance of making the years to come count. Fortunately for us, by the time we reach this phase we are likely to be extremely receptive to, and welcoming of positive, appropriately given advice. As a result, we are far less inclined to delay taking positive action and consequently far more likely to see faster results.

One of the secrets in making the most of our choices at mid-life is to be very conscious of the goals we want to pursue. For some of us, our primary concern may be to develop confidence in our bodies, which may feel physically sluggish and unfit; others may want most of all to improve the quality of poor diets; while many of us may feel that we want to pursue ways of boosting self-esteem. The main goal we need to have at the front of our minds is the need to focus with clarity and energy on the issues that are of prime concern to us. As long as we maintain this focus and make conscious positive choices we are likely to be constantly amazed at what it is possible for us to achieve.

However, before we move on to talk about specific ways of taking positive action towards these goals, we need to consider some of the basic assumptions from which we have to break free before we can move forward with confidence and vitality.

Rolling back the years: outmoded perspectives on menopause

The title of this book has been deliberately chosen to challenge many of the ideas that have previously been associated with menopause. Until relatively recently menopause was a taboo subject which was better left to itself, leaving many women silently struggling to find their own way through a confusing maze of experiences. At best, passing jokes might be made about hot flushes in order to try and defuse an embarrassing situation, but there was little in the way of positive advice available to us so that we could be empowered in managing our passage through this transition for ourselves.

One of the most important factors in challenging previous assumptions about mid-life experience for women is the impact of the baby boomers who are now moving through menopause. This generation of women has a reputation for not being afraid to challenge previous assumptions about the role that women could be expected to play within career structures, intimate relationships, and looking after their own health. As a result, the baby boomers have played a pivotal role in changing fundamental rules for women, emphasising the need for women to move beyond restrictive, sexist stereotypes into a future of greater personal freedom and self-expression.

We may now take the ground gained in the sixties and seventies as being par for the course because it all makes such good sense, and any other state of affairs would seem unthinkable. However, breaking any mould is often as painful as it is exhilarating, with the result that we should not forget the determination, resolve, and downright persistence it took in order to break free of well-established assumptions that at times bordered uncomfortably on naked prejudice.

One of the areas where baby boomers had an especially controversial role to play was challenging a male-dominated medical system when it came to women's health issues. From the seventies onwards, women began to play a more active role with regard to managing their own health, a desire which has been reflected in the publication of milestone books such as *Our Bodies, Ourselves*, written by the Boston Woman's Health Book Collective. Written very consciously as a health book for and by women right across the age spectrum, it provided a wealth of sound information about preventive measures for improving health, as well as up-to-date advice on diagnostic tests and treatment. Most significantly, this is a book that did not shy away from raising fundamental issues about the way women had previously been treated as patients and medical professionals by a male-dominated health system.

The positive impact of books such as this was enormous, with an explosion of information about self-care becoming available in the seventies, eighties, and continuing into the nineties. This coincided beautifully with a general boom in interest in non-conventional therapies which laid great emphasis on the need for preventive steps to be used as a way of protecting and maintaining optimum health.

This, in turn, created a climate where the idea of good health moved beyond a concept, popular in the fifties, of effective disease management with the appropriate 'magic bullet'. Instead of waging war on disease, a new perspective began to develop of the need to work in harmony with our own bodies in order to strengthen their self-regulating mechanisms. Within this context, more aggressive measures could be held in reserve for the situations that really demanded heroic treatment, with the added benefit that they were likely to be more effective when used sparingly and appropriately.

Now attention is being turned to menopause, with pertinent questions being asked about whether it is really appropriate to consider this as yet another disorder that needs treatment with an appropriate 'magic bullet'. In the case of menopause the drug of choice is considered to be HRT, given in whatever formula seems appropriate. However, the background in which HRT was developed gives us some important clues to the limitations and problems that may be associated with it as the sole tool at our disposal for managing menopause.

Sexual healing: early days of HRT

Oestrogen replacement therapy was hailed in the United States as an enormous breakthrough in keeping women youthful, sexually attractive and vital. This coincided with a decade when the majority of women would be defined by their roles as wives and mothers, with little chance of their having an opportunity to play any meaningful roles outside the home.

Any of the emancipation that had been gained for women during the wartime years, when they formed the basis of an essential workforce, was left behind by the fifties when the impetus was to get women back in their homes in order to allow men to return to the workplace. During this decade, being feminine was associated with the childbearing years, with scant attention being paid by men or women to the role they might hope to occupy beyond mid-life.

As a result, it is not too surprising if, as women found themselves drifting away from their fertile years, they would begin to panic, since they were approaching uncharted physical and emotional territory. What is worse, there would most likely be a general absence of positive role models to seek inspiration from. As a result, it appears that for many women, approaching the menopause was a fearful and distressing experience in the absence of any positive guidance to draw on when making this vital transition.

In addition, they had to contend with the unfairness of the existence of one set of rules for women and another for men. In other words, when a man began to show signs of grey hair and facial lines, these would be taken as outward indications of becoming more distinguished and powerful. On the other hand, visible signs of ageing in women such as greying hair and wrinkles would be interpreted in a completely contrasting way as evidence of a loss of personal power and identity. Within such a context the psychological pressure to mask signs of maturing would be overwhelming, since the consequences for a woman of showing her age would be to feel marginalised and threatened by younger women.

Within this context we can see why the promises held out by early forms of HRT might seem heaven-sent. These promises ranged from claims that HRT would rejuvenate skin tone, improve libido, counteract forgetfulness, stop hot flushes, and ease depression. Sadly, while some women did genuinely find that certain physical symptoms, such as hot flushes, dry skin and mucous membranes, did indeed respond favourably to treatment with HRT, they felt bereft and let down when they had to stop taking medication because of emerging health risks associated with long-term use. For some, symptoms returned with a vengeance once medication was stopped, and no advice was available that they could use to guide themselves through the deferred crisis.

For others there were even greater hurdles to overcome, since they may have been dismayed to find that HRT could not smooth over feelings of depression that were connected to confusion about identity, or grief over losing a central role as mother to a young family. In a situation such as this, instead of feeling a sense of exhilaration and achievement at having nurtured a growing family, and looking forward to developing fresh outlets for creative impulses and self-expression, there would be a tendency to feel that options had been closed off, with an attendant loss of confidence.

It is also noticeable that many of the early claims associated with using HRT pay as much attention to the age-defying, cosmetic aspects of treatment, as to its health-promoting aspects. There is also a subtle suggestion that by using HRT we may be given an opportunity to defer the ageing process by putting our biological clocks on hold. Questions rarely seemed to be asked about what lay on the other side of treatment, and how we might best plan for making this transition.

Seizing fresh opportunities: the alternative viewpoint

The alternative medical approach, on the other hand, takes a dynamic approach to health promotion, teaching patients how to explore strategies that support their experience of optimum health, rather than concentrating on the passive taking of pills in order to suppress symptoms of illness. From an alternative perspective, each person has an in-built, self-balancing mechanism that deals with problems as and when they arise for as long as the person remains in good health.

As a result, providing our systems are not overwhelmed by adverse stresses (these can be anything from psychological or physical stress to a severe viral illness), we tend to experience generally good health. On the other hand, once the system becomes overloaded by stress, troublesome symptoms can become established which refuse to shift without appropriate help and support.

At this point, it may be enough to rectify aspects of lifestyle that may be challenging an already compromised system in order to re-establish basic equilibrium. This could include improving a poor diet, reducing alcohol consumption, exploring relaxation techniques, or reducing an overly challenging workload. If this is not enough, then it may be necessary to prescribe a course of appropriate alternative treatment that could include Chinese or Western medical herbalism, acupuncture, or homoeopathy.

Whatever course of alternative medical intervention is adopted, it will be basically aimed at strengthening the body to deal with the problem itself. As a result, medicines are believed to work in harmony with the body's own efforts, rather than temporarily blocking or suppressing what the body is attempting to do. Effective treatment should also result in improvements being experienced within the system as a whole, rather than some symptoms being improved at the expense of others, or a stream of side effects being initiated that demand yet more treatment.

Perhaps most importantly of all, alternative systems of healing such as homoeopathy benefit the mind, emotions and body in equal measure. Many physical symptoms are seen as being linked to emotional stress, or repressed trauma, with the result that substantial benefits are often to be seen initially on a mental and emotional level. Once this is well established, physical problems are seen to recede to a corresponding degree.

Well, we might ask, this all sounds terrific, but what does it have to do with menopause? In reality, the alternative approach to stimulating optimum health has an enormous amount to contribute to any discussion of how we approach, and move through and beyond mid-life. Unlike the conventional medical perspective which attempts to trick the body into believing that hormone levels are not substantially changing by supplementing oestrogen and progesterone when required, alternative medical approaches attempt to support the body in accomplishing this major transition as efficiently and swiftly as possible.

Since effective alternative therapy also has the huge advantage of stimulating energy levels and increasing overall vitality, this often has the desirable knock-on effect of making positive change in lifestyle more achievable. This, in turn, often has the positive effect of boosting self-confidence and self-esteem which are invaluable commodities at mid-life and beyond.

The importance of balance

If we had to isolate the philosophical thread running through all of the major alternative medical therapies, it must be the fundamental need to restore optimum balance on mental, emotional and physical levels for each individual patient. The interdependence of psychological and physical health cannot be stressed too much for an alternative therapist, with the major systems of the body working as a complex network of checks and balances.

If an imbalance arises in one area, this has a 'domino effect', often resulting in a corresponding series of imbalances occurring elsewhere. As a result, if we attend to only one aspect of imbalance without considering the effect on the body as a whole, there is unlikely to be a general change for the better. If we add into the equation that most conventional drugs also have undesirable side effects, the result can often be even less satisfactory.

If we consider the process of menopause and the changes that lead up to it, this can be a particularly illuminating example of the exciting opportunities alternative treatment can offer us. As we shall see in the following chapter, a naturally occurring menopause is not a sudden event which descends on us overnight. It is the cumulative effect of a number of natural subtle changes that take place in our hormonal balance over an extended period of time. This process can be speeded up, slowed down, or made less or more intense according to a series of factors. These could include our genetic inheritance, the quality of our diets, the amount of conventional medicine that we have taken, or the amount of stress that we have to deal with on a day-to-day basis.

We also need to bear in mind that a naturally occurring menopause does not form a watershed beyond which oestrogen secretion stops abruptly. For those of us who have a reasonably stable and healthy body weight and who are generally in sound health, oestrogen secretion continues at a reduced output, until it slowly diminishes to its slight cruising level. If this process happens at a naturally slow pace, symptoms should not be distressingly traumatic or extended over a dauntingly long period of time.

If we consider that the strength of alternative therapies lies in their ability to re-establish equilibrium as smoothly and swiftly as possible in our systems as a whole, we can see that there is enormous potential for them to provide us with vital help in making the transition involved in the ongoing process of menopause as painlessly as possible. We can regard this balancing action on unstable, see-sawing hormone levels as being a mirror image of the help that many of us may have gained from alternative therapies in dealing with troublesome symptoms connected with pre-menstrual tension.

Many of these symptoms echo problems that occur in relation to menopause such as fluid retention, mood swings, recurrent headaches, and breast tenderness. In the same way that alternative therapies can even out our experience of pre-menstrual problems by encouraging hormonal secretions to work in as balanced a way as possible in times of flux, the same therapeutic approach can support our bodies in coming to terms with hormonal fluctuations at menopause.

It helps if we remember that the internal upheaval of menopause continues for a limited time, and provided we have appropriate medical support to get through the phase of transition as uneventfully as possible, we are free to reach a point of welcome stasis at the other side. Fluctuations may still occur, even at this point, but with adequate therapeutic help and positive advice about lifestyle changes that will help us move on, we should find that we can reclaim our lives once again.

A fresh perspective on the value of symptoms

As a homoeopath, I am very aware that the alternative medical response to the nature of symptoms is quite different from that of a conventional physician. Orthodox doctors regard symptoms as invaluable indicators that point them in the direction of the most appropriate diagnosis. This tentative diagnosis can be further confirmed by conducting appropriate tests. Once the disease has been confirmed, treatment can be decided upon, since selection of orthodox drugs is made according to whatever disease condition has been identified.

Alternative practitioners, on the other hand, work from the premise that whatever treatment is selected must not only correspond to the symptoms that the patient is suffering from, but must also match the sensations of ill-health experienced by that patient as a unique individual. In addition, symptoms are seen in an essentially benign light as the body's way of communicating to us that all is not well. If they are persistently ignored, there is every chance that they will get increasingly strong until we have no choice but to take positive action.

When we don't pay attention to the early warning signs that symptoms provide us with, it is rather like ignoring a warning light flashing on the dashboard of a car. If we ignore the flashing light for long enough, we can be sure that the car will eventually grind to a halt and won't be able to perform well again until the underlying problem has been rectified.

The same is true of our bodies: if we refuse to eat the best quality diet (the equivalent of using top-grade petrol) we aren't likely to feel full of vitality, and will run out of stream very quickly. The saying 'if you don't use it you lose it' is as true of our bodies as it is of our cars. Appropriate physical demands will beneficially work our hearts, muscles and joints, in the same way that our cars will seize up and their batteries go flat if they are left idle for too long.

Apart from the main presenting symptoms that we can use to diagnose what category of illness a patient is suffering from, alternative therapists are interested in more subtle changes that a conventional physician would not find so relevant. So, for example, if a patient came for homoeopathic treatment of hot flushes and night sweats, they would not just be asked to give a detailed account of what made the flushes better or worse, or how long-lasting they were. They would also be questioned closely about their emotional health, general energy levels, and their ability to deal effectively with stress.

In addition, they might be asked to give a run-down of their daily eating patterns, paying special attention to the quality of their diet. Details of general medical history are also relevant since they can reveal any inherited patterns of illness that may cause problems in the future.

The aim behind building up this very personal medical profile is to allow the therapist to select a form of treatment that will restore that individual to optimum health at all levels, rather than selecting a drug that is specifically designed to target hot flushes and night sweats alone. We could argue that that is precisely what a GP would be setting out to do by prescribing HRT, which claims to have a beneficially broader-based action than just reducing the frequency and severity of hot flushes. On the other hand, as we shall see from Chapter 6, 'The Pros and Cons of Hormone Replacement Therapy', HRT brings with it a series of side effects that can outweigh the potential benefits.

2

Understanding Menopause

For many women the word menopause has a loaded emotional charge, a charge that has been made more intense by everyone from the medical establishment to the media. So far, a great deal of the emphasis has been on menopause as a period in a woman's life that signifies an ending and a sad farewell to the positive advantages that are conferred upon the young. This image is vigorously bolstered by the acting profession and advertising companies, who reserve attractive parts for young, nubile females with model-like bodies. It is apparently almost impossible for women over forty to land roles in Hollywood that portray a middle-aged actress as sexy, attractive and exciting. It is understood instead that if they wait a little longer, they are likely to be cast as safe, motherly, rather eccentric characters.

If we also consider that much of the information obtained from a conventional medical source tends to focus on the problems that can be associated with menopause (osteoporosis, heart disease, urinary tract infections, and changes in moisture levels in the skin and mucous membranes), is it any wonder that we are likely to feel apprehensive, depressed and downright fearful as we think about reaching menopausal age? It is also interesting to consider that the main treatment on offer from conventional doctors is hormone replacement therapy (HRT), which in theory delays the speed at which our bodies come to terms with the fundamental change that is taking place in the time leading up to and during menopause.

Positive perspectives on menopause

We are quite correct to ask the basic question at this point: 'Does it really have to be this way?' The answer is a resounding 'No'. There are encouragingly wide, exciting and effective options open to us as we manage our menopause that are outlined in the course of the following chapters of this book. There is no pretence made that experiencing menopause may not be challenging, frustrating and problematic at times, but attention is also drawn to the fact that there are practical strategies for dealing with difficult situations as they arise.

In addition, the important message is also communicated that menopause is not a disease state or pathological condition, but an inevitable major transitional experience that all women will experience in their middle years. It will come as a breath of fresh air to many that menopause does not necessarily have to involve a host of gruesome symptoms that turn our lives upside down. After all, a significant proportion of women will go through this rite of passage under their own steam with the minimum of discomfort and distress. Apart from sheer good luck, the following factors appear to also play a part in predisposing us towards a smoother passage through menopause:

- The experience of close female relatives (mothers, aunts and grandmothers) may have some bearing on the age at which we go through menopause and the severity of symptoms that we may experience. In other words, if our mothers and grandmothers had a pretty trouble-free and generally uneventful experience of menopause, we have a better than fighting chance that we may be just as fortunate, especially if we are aware of simple steps we can take in preparation for this event.
- Avoiding smoking can also have an impact on the age at which we experience symptoms. It has been suggested that smokers

will have on average an earlier menopause than non-smokers, due to the negative effect of smoking on oestrogen secretion.

- Those of us who have a stable weight pattern, not having gone through periods of crash dieting where we have been significantly underweight, are likely to suffer less severe symptoms. This is linked to the way in which adequate body fat reserves have a part to play in oestrogen production. Those of us who are very slightly above our desired body weight may have a considerably less troubled experience as a result.

- Our expectations may also play a larger part than we realise in shaping the menopausal experience we have. If we are uneasy with our bodies and have a very negative expectation of what may be ahead of us (possibly communicated to us by close female relatives or friends), this appears to have a genuinely less than positive impact on the experience we actually have. This may be linked with the way that approaching the menopause with fear and dread is likely to have a powerful effect in raising our overall stress levels. This, in turn, can result in our adrenal glands becoming overworked and depleted. When this happens it has the undesirable knock-on effect of predisposing us to obvious extra symptoms of hormone imbalance – something we can well do without in our pre-menopausal years when hormone levels will be fluctuating of their own accord.

Before we explore more general issues connected with menopause, however, it will be helpful to take a straight look at the facts of the most basic issues in connection with this major change in our lives. This way we will really understand what we are dealing with when we talk about menopause.

All you wanted to know about menopause and were afraid to ask!

What exactly is the menopause?

Strictly speaking, the menopause has occurred when we have had our last menstrual period. As a result, we can't really know that it has happened for sure, until we have been period-free for at least a year or more. This is why it is suggested that even though we may be confident that our periods have ended, we should still use contraceptive measures for approximately two years after our last period. Factually speaking, once we have gone through the menopause we no longer have the capacity to bear children, and the time of onset of the menopause is largely determined by the productive life of our ovaries. Once they cease their normal pattern of functioning we will experience menopausal symptoms. Some of us may be puzzled by the use of the term 'climacteric' and wonder how on earth this relates to the menopause. The meaning of climacteric begins to become clear if we consider it as matching the period of puberty that happens at the other end of the age spectrum. In other words, the climacteric can be seen as a mirror image of the years that make up adolescence or puberty, when the ovaries begin to mature and carry out the function that nature intended. As a result, the climacteric may be used as a term that encompasses an ongoing phase when ovarian function and hormonal secretions decline. This phase may continue for a long as fifteen to twenty years and encompasses the pre-, peri-, and post-menopausal stages.

What leads up to it?

It is important to realise that pre-menopausal changes (also referred to as peri-menopause when describing the stage either side of the last menstrual period) may take several years to develop. In a naturally occurring pre-menopause, changes may be so subtle that very little attention is paid to them (this may especially be the case in those of us who have a history of pre-menstrual syndrome), since many symptoms may overlap such as mood swings, an increase in fluid retention, sleep disturbance and fatigue. Additional problems that may arise at this time include hot flushes, night sweats, dryness of mucous membranes (dryness of the eyes and vaginal tissues may be especially noticeable), a tendency to frequent urinary tract infections, recurrent headaches, migraines, lowered libido, itchy skin, and periods that change their pattern.

The varying patterns of periods that were once as regular as clockwork can be rather bewildering to start with, until we catch on to what is happening. This is especially the case if we experience an early peri-menopause which may rather take us by surprise. Possible changes in pattern may include any of the following:

- Periods become more frequent, heavier and more painful:
- Bleeding happens at roughly a twenty-eight-day cycle but is so heavy that it becomes difficult to provide adequate sanitary protection (especially at night when tampons and towels may need to be changed every hour or so).
- Periods become lighter and less predictable in onset until they slowly phase themselves out.
- Periods may suddenly stop.
- Periods may appear to have stopped for a year or so, and then suddenly reappear.

When does it happen?

The age at which menopause can be expected to occur will vary from one woman to another, but on average we can expect it to happen around the age of fifty-one. In theory, menopause can occur any time between the age of forty-five and fifty-five, but in more unusual cases it can happen in the early forties or late fifties. For general guidelines on factors that may influence time of onset and severity of menopausal symptoms see the section on 'Positive perspectives on menopause' above (p. 19). As a general rule, the time of onset may be influenced by general quality of lifestyle including nutritional status as well as inherited factors. As a result, we may be correct to assume that the healthier our general lifestyle is, the later our menopause may occur.

All of the above relates to a naturally occurring menopause that sets in under its own steam. However, we should also consider factors that can induce a premature menopause (before the age of forty). These include the following:

- Surgical removal of the reproductive organs as a result of hysterectomy. If the ovaries are left intact, menopause will still occur at younger age than it would without surgical intervention, but this will be later than cases where the ovaries are removed.
- Chemotherapy or radiation treatment in order to treat cancer.
- Diseases that involve an auto-immune reaction, where the body can't distinguish between an undesirable invader and its own tissues. Examples of auto-immune diseases include lupus and rheumatoid arthritis. Although not in itself an auto-immune disorder, mumps can also damage the ovaries if the disease occurs in adult women (in the same way that the testicles may be at risk in adult males).
- A history of eating disorders (anorexia nervosa or bulimia nervosa) or a punishing exercise regime with strict dietary control may also adversely affect oestrogen production leading to a disrupted menstrual history and early menopause. Great care should be taken in these situations to assess bone density, since these are also significant co-factors in increasing our risk of developing osteoporosis.

What can we realistically expect?

However sobering and unsettling the lists of symptoms given above might seem, it is extremely important to bear in mind that not all of these problems are likely to occur together, and if we take steps to protect our health, there is a fighting chance that we will accomplish this major change in our lives with the minimum amount of trauma and fuss. It helps to bear in mind that not all women experience major symptoms, and many appear to sail through menopause without so much as a backward glance. For those of us who begin to struggle with hot flushes and disturbed sleep pattern, there is an increasingly helpful amount of advice available that can support us through these challenges (see Chapter 7, 'Alternative Self-Help for Short-Term Symptoms'). Alternatively, if concerns about osteoporosis and/or heart disease are causing anxiety and you want to put available methods of treatment in a balanced context, see Chapter 6, 'The Pros and Cons of Hormone Replacement Therapy'.

Above all else, never forget that those of us who experience a naturally occurring climacteric will have plenty of time within which to adjust to the changes that our bodies are experiencing. After all, it has been estimated that the whole process can take anything up to fifteen to twenty years. The vital quality that appears to be most important in supporting ourselves through this transitional phase of life is one of understanding what is happening at each stage. This is, of course, likely to be different for everyone, since each of us will have our own individual experience of menopause. However, it helps to know about certain predictable symptoms that can arise, to which we have a wide range of practical solutions.

Above all else, if we understand what is happening to us we are less likely to feel fearful and anxious, as well as more empowered to take positive action. By turning the tables in this way, we are far less likely to feel distanced from, or at odds with what our bodies are trying to do. Considering alternative and complementary strategies for supporting us through this transition is especially important, since therapies such as homoeopathy, Western medical herbalism, and traditional Chinese medicine appear to work by stimulating and supporting the body in accomplishing what it is attempting to do as swiftly and efficiently as possible. As a result, when symptoms disappear they are far less likely to return than they might in response to conventional medicine, which usually works by temporarily suppressing or dampening down symptoms. This is why, once conventional medication is discontinued, symptoms can make an unwelcome reappearance since the body has not been strengthened to come to terms with its underlying predisposition to the problem itself.

Puberty as a mirror image of menopause

Considering menopause as a parallel rite of passage to puberty can do a great deal to positively modify our view of menopausal changes and symptoms. If we have come to fear what follows menopause as a series of disease symptoms that inevitably need medical treatment, it can be extremely liberating to consider that all of us will have already have come through an equally turbulent life crisis at puberty. Although the onset of regular periods and the physical maturing of our bodies may not bring attendant concerns about osteoporosis and heart disease, there are plenty of health problems that could be seen to be associated with puberty if we chose to look on it that way.

Eating disorders, pre-menstrual symptoms, and general problems associated with confusion about identity are all possibilities once puberty is well under way. However, it would be very unusual to consider puberty as a medical crisis that demands disease-management techniques in order for a young woman to make a successful transition to womanhood. Most of us will regard our bodies as being basically equipped to cope with this major shift in hormonal balance, provided we are in generally good health.

We could correctly say that we are given a powerful introduction to the roles that sex hormones play with regard to our emotional, mental and physical health and well-being when we reach the age of about eleven. This is the predictable age at which girls begin to experience the physical changes of puberty which involve enlargement of the breasts, and the growth of body hair. Once these are in evidence, we can be sure that the first period will appear before too long. In the same way that the timing of menopause is variable, although the average age of onset of puberty is around eleven, some girls may experience much earlier changes around the age of eight or nine, while others may experience a late onset around thirteen or fourteen.

Just as periods take some time before they settle down to a regular and predictable cycle at puberty, menopausal women are also likely to find that their periods become irregular and unpredictable as they are phasing themselves out. We can see an important parallel between both ends of the age spectrum as our bodies are striving to stabilise hormone levels in order to reach an optimum healthy level. Both processes take time to develop, often causing temporary havoc before they reach a desirable point of stasis.

Once we hit puberty, the cells in our ovaries begin to secrete oestrogens which form the primary group of female sex hormones and which are responsible for the development of visible secondary sexual characteristics such as growth of the breasts and widening of the hips. Non-visible changes also take place through the action of oestrogens in the womb and vagina.

However, although most of us are aware of the importance of the action of oestrogen at puberty and menopause, fewer of us may consider the essential role played by androgens which are secreted by the adrenal glands. Without adequate secretion of androgens we would not experience the growth spurt that characteristically takes place at puberty. Although androgens are primarily considered to be male hormones (they include testosterone), they must be present in a balanced way in the female body as well for a healthy hormonal balance to exist. As a result, once we enter the peri-menopausal phase, the balance of androgens is changed along with the amount of female sex hormones secreted by the body.

However, physical similarities apart, there are more important psychological parallels that we can see between puberty and menopause if we look carefully enough at the emotional charge that can surround each of these major transitional experiences. Both events can be regarded as traumatic and inevitable rites of passage that potentially involve pain, confusion, and unwillingness to leave one phase of life behind and move on to another. The latter may be made even more difficult and traumatic if we consciously or unconsciously perceive the next phase to be full of insecurity, unknown challenges, and fear.

At puberty we experience an overpowering biological impetus propelling us toward adulthood and rapidly developing sexual maturity. On the other hand, this powerful force that is bearing us forward can sometimes come in conflict with a marked desire to hold on to the past security of childhood with its compensations of freedom from responsibility. When these conflicting forces meet each other, the common problems of eating disorders, confusion, extreme mood swings, painful lack of confidence, fatigue, pre-menstrual syndrome, depression, introversion, and lack of motivation can make themselves painfully apparent.

Issues of conflict

At menopause we can experience a very similar clash of interests. This is often set in motion by the powerful tension between the desire to hold on to the security and familiarity of the years when we are treated as being sexually attractive and fertile (this is one of the striking features of living in a society where images of sexual attractiveness are intimately bound up with remaining young and nubile), and the biological imperative which pushes us inevitably towards a phase where certain basic options such as childbearing are no longer available to us. Symptoms that can be regarded as emerging from this conflict include flagging libido, problems with intimacy, depression, lack of vitality, anxiety, and confusion about identity.

Both menopause and puberty involve a basic need to break with the past, so that we are free to move on to a greater sense of independence with a renewed sense of identity and self-esteem. In order to do this successfully we have to come to terms with, and resolve our inner conflicts as well as giving others the opportunity and understanding space within which they can work through their own conflicting expectations of us. Many of us feel great frustration when we are given the impression that we should be conforming to some sort of stereotype of meno-pausal woman.

The latter should be resisted at all costs, since it can blunt the growing sense of exhilaration and excitement that many of us come to feel when we discover an essential freedom that comes with the menopause: the powerful freedom of being ourselves for the first time. However, this is only given a chance to flourish if we stop looking backwards and denying the ageing process, and avoid desperately trying to suppress the changes that it inevitably brings along as part of the deal. On the other hand, it is vitally important to stress that this does not suggest that we adopt an approach which passively accepts an encroaching decline in our personal power, dynamism and attractiveness. On the contrary, it should be much more of a positive acceptance and acknowledgment of a natural development that requires appropriate support, guidance, and access to the most reliable medical information in order to help us reach a point of optimum mental, emotional and physical balance beyond menopause.

The unspoken assumption is also often made that those of us who may have chosen not to have children may have a more difficult experience than those of us who are mothers. However, this does not appear to be automatically the case by any means. Those of us who are fulfilled in our close relationships, who have also developed a satisfying and challenging career, and who are in fine emotional, mental and physical health, have an excellent chance of making the most of the years through menopause. Even when we have left our careers behind, there is a very strong chance that we will retain absorbing interests if we have the energy levels that come from a healthy constitution and positive support from a network of close relationships.

On the other hand, if we have taken our primary identity and motivation from being a mother, there is a very strong chance that we may have some hefty issues to deal with at menopause. Those of us who have chosen to juggle career demands with the challenges of being a mother may also discover that we have had too little time to care for ourselves, with the unfortunate consequence that we may feel emotionally, mentally and physically exhausted by the time we are approaching menopause.

Although these are rather extreme scenarios, they are given with the intention of highlighting the primary importance of protecting and preserving optimum levels of health. This is often a much stronger factor in determining our experience of menopause than if we have decided to have children or not. After all, we are all individuals who will respond to our individual circumstances in our own individual way. However, the gift of positive health is a factor of central importance in determining how well we cope with the life choices that we make.

Positive aspects of menopause

Many of us will be very well versed by now about the pitfalls and negative side of menopause, but few of us may have been encouraged to see any desirable features that may be associated with it. After all, how many of us are encouraged to consider any of the positive sides of moving beyond this major watershed in life? Since we don't have much choice one way or another about putting off this process indefinitely, surely it is time to contemplate some of the changes that may prove to change our lives for the better?

One of the most welcome changes associated with post-menopausal years is the absence of periods for the first time since puberty (apart, of course for the odd nine months during pregnancy). I have yet to meet a woman who is not delighted that at last they are freed from the discomfort and paraphernalia involved in having a period every month. How many of us would not welcome being able to plan a holiday or special event at short notice, knowing that we don't even have to think about whether we are having a period or not at that time? Also consider the common symptoms of PMS that are too often part and parcel of the roller-coaster ride leading up to the onset of each period. How many of us would not wish to be free of unpredictable mood swings, breast tenderness, fluid retention and abdominal cramps? The positive reaction to leaving periods behind is also one of the main reasons why many women do not react well to HRT, since this often involves returning to a situation of a monthly bleed.

Freedom from contraception is also one of greatest joys to most post-menopausal women. When we consider the complications of choosing an effective and appropriate form of contraception that suits us, our sexual partners, and our individual circumstances, surely it is something to be celebrated when we can dispense with this as a relevant issue? Many of us find that we discover the joy of an uninhibited and spontaneous sex life for the first time as we move beyond menopause. This is not only linked to the absence of anxieties about unwanted pregnancy, but also has a great deal to do with the way in which we may be enjoying an increased amount of privacy during our middle years. This particularly applies to women who chose to have their children in their late twenties and thirties: they are likely to find that they experience menopause around the time their children have made independent lives for themselves away from home. Once this transitory phase has been accomplished and come to terms with, many of us may be delighted by the new-found privacy and change of pace of life that we experience.

If we are in a long-term relationship we may also find that we have moved through menopause at the same time that our partner has taken retirement. Challenging as this can be for both partners, it can also provide us with a vital opportunity for greater understanding and emotional intimacy. Time which had previously been in very short supply and at a premium may suddenly be more flexible and available. This can provide us with the valuable incentive that we need to start new directions in life, pursuing personal or professional interests that may have been put on the back burner for a long time.

Menopause can also provide us with an essential change of perspective once we have moved through to the other side of it. So many complex questions arise in connection with women's biological clocks. Should we have children? If we do, how can this be combined with a career structure? If we have a child, how do we feel about 'only' children, and when is the right time to consider having more? How do we feel about taking sole responsibility for our children if we are not in a stable relationship? What impact is having a child going to have on a long-term relationship? What are the financial repercussions likely to be?

However, once we have experienced menopause these questions will have been answered for us one way or another, with the positive result that many of us may feel empowered to move forward to a new phase of our lives. Of course, as with any other choice that we may make in life, there are bound to be some regrets and a feeling that we might, with the advantage of hindsight, have chosen to do some things differently. But, as with so many challenging experiences in life, when we have confronted an event which may have involved a great deal of anticipatory anxiety, once it is behind us we often feel a huge sense of relief. It is also true that having too many options open to us at any one time can have the effect of being rather draining of energy, and once some of these options become redundant or inappropriate, we can concentrate in a focused way on our obvious course of action.

Moving with the flow

It is generally acknowledged that if we brace ourselves in a state of denial and go kicking and screaming against any inevitable change we are likely to end up feeling drained, depressed, disempowered and demoralised. However, if in practical terms we do as much as we can to ensure as positive an outcome as possible in the face of upheaval, and try to move as harmoniously as possible with the direction in which the change is taking us, the outcome is likely to be far more satisfying and positive. This is far from a suggestion that we should become passive in the face of a challenging situation, but more that we should put our energies into 'going with the flow' rather than unrealistically obstructing it.

Nowhere is this more true than when we contemplate the years approaching and directly following the menopause. If we take appropriate action to prepare ourselves for this challenge we are likely to develop a greater intuitive understanding and practical knowledge of the state of our bodies, minds and emotions. When we are armed in this way we will be in the best position possible to explore the practical steps open to us in supporting ourselves through any difficulties that may arise.

Taking action

Perhaps the greatest ally in supporting us through changes leading up to, and following the menopause is the saying already mentioned: 'If you don't use it you lose it'. This applies to what we do with our bodies and minds as we approach and move beyond menopause if we want to give ourselves the best chance of enjoying optimum energy levels, maximum fitness, an enduring sex life, mental clarity and a sense of emotional well-being. By starting an appropriate programme of physical fitness we can maximise our chances of keeping a strong, supple body while giving ourselves essential protection against developing osteoporosis. Remaining mentally active by involvement in professional challenges is of vital importance in keeping us intellectually sharp, while keeping sexually active is a vital ally in maintaining our sense of ourselves as sensual beings, as well as making an important contribution towards protecting the health of our sexual organs.

The benefits of discovering the joy of exercise are especially important when we reach mid-life. Although there are undoubtable advantages in being physically fit when we are in our twenties, they are not the sort to be immediately obvious without a series of fairly intricate lab tests. However, once we reach our fifties and beyond, the benefits become more obvious with each decade that goes by. It has been suggested that while regular exercise can improve a youthful body by approximately 10 per cent, it can benefit an older person by as much as 50 per cent. These positive effects were highlighted by a recent study involving post-menopausal women at Tufts University Centre on Ageing in Boston, which revealed that those who became involved in a strength training programme for a year reversed the course of their ageing by anything between fifteen and twenty years. Benefits included increased bone and muscle mass, lowered heart rate and more toned body shape.

However, it helps to bear in mind that whenever we talk about exercise it needs to be appropriate to our individual needs and temperaments. While we may have enjoyed high-impact, punishing aerobics classes in our twenties and thirties, this approach is likely to be positively disadvantageous to us in our fifties and beyond. Not only does pounding away on a hard surface put enormous stress and pressure on vulnerable knee and ankle joints, but it can also contribute towards the face looking drawn and exhausted. In addition, an overly-harsh, high-impact approach can also leave our bodies looking too spare and sinewy. On the other hand, an appropriate combination of stretching, weight training, and relaxation can have discernible rejuvenating and revitalising benefits.

One of the best ways of preparing ourselves for an active approach to this major transition in our lives is to consider that this is a marvellous time to pause and take stock of our lives so far. It has been suggested that mid-life provides us with a tremendous opportunity for gaining a clear perspective on what has happened to us so far, so that we can make maximum use of the time ahead. If we consider menopause in this light we can see how it can mark the beginning of an important time of change and renewal rather than becoming a potent symbol of the fear of ageing and closure.

As we have mentioned at the beginning of this chapter, it helps a great deal to remember that our expectations can have a powerful effect on the outcome of any significant event. This is especially true of menopause, since there is evidence to suggest that if we expect to become weak, unwell and vulnerable in mind and body, there is a good chance that this negative expectation may become self-fulfilling. On the other hand, if we identify with powerful role models who are healthy, energetic, positive, confident, and attractive well into their sixties and beyond, this positive expectation can also become self-fulfilling.

Detailed advice is given in the next few chapters on how we can tailor aspects of our lifestyle to best prepare us for, and move beyond, menopause. These include sections on eating for maximum health, choosing a physical fitness plan that suits us, and ways of setting new goals for ourselves so that we feel empowered by this challenging time in our lives.

3

Mind over Matter: Preparation for Menopause

We may not know it, but our minds are one of the most powerful anti-ageing allies we have at our disposal. Our mental and emotional equilibrium can also play a pivotal role in determining the experience of overall health and vitality that we enjoy on a daily basis. Sounds too good to be true doesn't it?

In other words, before we even consider the extra help we can draw on from alternative and conventional medical sources, from improvements in nutrition, and judicious amounts of exercise, we already have a formidable health-enhancing tool closer to hand within our own minds. The trick, of course, is in learning how to make full use of this extraordinary potential by consciously activating our own inbuilt capacity for stress reduction. In order to do this, we need to understand which of the changes in lifestyle that are available to us are health-promoting, and which are anything but.

At no other phase of our lives is this quite so important as when we are approaching menopause. These are the years when we are likely to be more aware than at any other time of the way in which our bodies, emotions and minds are going through a range of perceptible changes.

If we fail to understand how these are natural and predictable aspects of an ongoing process, we are likely to respond with fear or an overwhelming sense of denial. Sadly, both of these unconscious strategies will make our situation more difficult, since negative stress appears to play a major role in aggravating menopausal problems.

On the other hand, the important positive news is that the reverse is also true. In other words, if we understand and work with the direction in which our bodies, minds and emotions are moving, we can do an enormous amount to support ourselves through this transitional phase while at the same time unlocking our potential for health and vitality beyond mid-life.

Forever young or forever healthy?

Before we go any further in discussing the tools we have at our disposal in order to secure a flourishing mid-life, it would help at this point to establish what our main priorities are.

The information that follows is primarily designed to help us become healthy and as full of vitality as our individual optimum level of energy allows us to. If we want to boost our basic level of self-esteem with such additional means as hair colour, make-up, the latest skin-care and fashions, this is fine. On the other hand, if we have instinctively been longing to follow Germaine Greer's advice to release and embrace the crone inside of us, and if that feels good for us, that's equally fine.

The secret is for each of us to discover where our own optimum state of balance and equilibrium lies, so that we feel focused, liberated and positive. If we put all of our efforts into pursuing an unrealistic goal of permanent youth without attending to the deeper issues of becoming truly well, the chances are that we will become eventually deeply disappointed, and possibly downright depressed. Extreme measures such as radical cosmetic surgery, rigid diets, and punishing exercise plans may seem to work for a limited amount of time, but they become their own prison in the long term.

Even more strikingly, if all we do is attend to the surface by making modifications through corrective surgery, it appears that we relatively soon return to square one if we have ignored deeper issues that are crying out for change. So, for instance, if we feel that we are unhappy with carrying excess inches around our abdomens or upper thighs and have it removed by surgical means, in the short term we may be delighted at the results. However, if we haven't made adjustments in our daily eating plans or made a concerted effort to get physically fit, we won't have corrected the situation in the long term.

The same can also be true of facial surgery, since concentrating on eliminating a superficial flaw is not likely to be the key to correcting our self-esteem. Instead, we are more likely to find an alternative focus of imperfection in another area of our body. Once we adopt this route as the solution to our problems, we are unlikely to reach a point where we are completely satisfied.

On the other hand, if we adopt an 'I-may-just-as-well-let-it-all-hang-out' approach because it seems too late to make a difference, this is unlikely to lead us towards a positive state of balance and self-esteem either. Not doing anything because of feeling negative about ourselves can be just as much of a problem as pursuing the course of constant corrective surgery described above. The crux of the issue is that both can spring from a negative self-image which needs addressing if genuinely balanced health is to be experienced on mental, emotional and physical levels.

The key to finding and maintaining the necessary balance lies in recognising that change is an integral part of life: if we try to freeze-frame ourselves as we were in our thirties we are sure to come to grief. On the other hand, once we appreciate that we are moving on and celebrate the way this can release us from the past, while we can still hang on to the benefits that hard-won experience has taught us, the future takes on an exciting colouring. Balance is not achieved by rushing towards becoming old before our time, any more than it is gained by expending huge amounts of energy and money in denying that important years have passed by.

Balance is achieved when we feel we are at a point where we

welcome the opportunities that are presented to us as a result of change, and have the mental and emotional flexibility to seize them, as well as enough physical energy to carry plans through. It is noticeable that those of us who develop this perspective are the ones who appear to be eternally youthful. This is a precious quality that does not fade with time since it comes from within, rather than being dependent on the results of purely superficial measures. As we have seen above, the latter will only give short-lived satisfaction if we depend on them to solve our internal problems.

In the next section we will be exploring the common features possessed by those who remain genuinely youthful, followed by a general run-down of positive lifestyle changes that will support us in making the most of our potential for mental, emotional and physical balance through effective stress-reduction. After all, whatever path we choose must lead us towards good health as our first priority. Once we take the steps that are appropriate to us and we experience how it feels to be positively well rather than just being free of symptoms of disease, we are likely to be amazed at the positive benefits that emerge.

You are as old as you feel

Trite as this phrase must sound, there is growing evidence to suggest that there is more truth in it than we might have initially thought. Our expectations of the ageing process appear to have a major impact on our experience of emotional and physical health as we move beyond menopause. Of course, our expectations aren't the only issue with regard to how we age, since our genetic inheritance and general quality of life (including everything from the viability of our closest relationships to the nature of our daily diets) will have a huge impact on the rate and the way in which our bodies adjust to getting older.

However, it has been suggested that there are certain attitudes which are common features of those who have been christened the 'superyoung' or 'ultra agers'. These are people who genuinely appear to be younger than their actual age. These mental and emotional attitudes cannot stop the ageing process in its tracks, or change our genetic inheritance. On the other hand, adopting some of the following psychological strategies may do more to keep us genuinely youthful than the most expensive anti-wrinkle cream that money can buy!

Flexibility

One of the most powerful attributes of those who are genuinely youthful is the gift of adapting to change. Conversely, the hallmark of those who are old before their time is the marked tendency to brace themselves against any change, however small. This leads to a huge amount of energy and vitality being fruitlessly wasted in trying to control the uncontrollable. If, however, we can learn how to move with good grace in whatever direction inevitable change is taking us, the chances are that we will begin to feel unexpectedly relieved and liberated. Even better, we may begin to enjoy the challenges that are brought by change in our lives, instead of constantly being threatened by it. This is especially important, since it has been suggested by Dr David Weeks (author of *Superyoung*) that our rate of ageing may be accelerated by feelings of anxiety, resentment and anger.

Curiosity

Those who are genuinely youthful never lose their sense of curiosity about the world around them. A loss of interest in events and people around us can be an indication of early signs of depression, and it is often a precursor of our withdrawing emotionally and physically from others. On the other hand, if we continue to be healthily curious, we will be inclined to interact with others, giving ourselves the basic stimulation that we all need if we are to avoid becoming mentally and emotionally stagnant.

Remaining socially active

As we get older some of us may instinctively retreat, feeling that it is too late to have a social life. We may claim that this is because we are too tired, too jaded, or that we have just got out of the habit through focusing on our professional or domestic commitments. The hardest part is usually getting ourselves moving in the first place, since it can be nerve-wracking to be faced with social interaction if we are out of practice. However, it really is worth the effort, since the benefits of refusing to be solitary are well worth fighting for.

These include a greater possibility of keeping problems in perspective if we interact with others. After all, there is nothing as likely to give us an unbalanced sense of our problems than constantly going over them in our own heads. On the other hand, once we are able to talk them over with a good friend, our perspective changes straight away. Being part of a social network can also provide us with an important sense that there is a world going on outside the confines of our own homes. Not only is this a focus of positive stimulation, but it also provides an important balancing factor so that issues connected to our home environment can be viewed within a broader context.

One of the best ways of becoming socially active after a period of inactivity is to enrol on a course that we may have been putting off for various reasons. This can have a double advantage, since pursuing a new interest will give us fresh mental stimulation while also introducing us to a new circle of people. This, in turn, can lead to all sorts of fresh interests and developments, provided we remain open to what life has to offer us.

Staying productive

Feeling we have a useful contribution to make is one of the key factors in keeping us youthful. Having a significant professional role to play has a particularly positive impact on women as they move beyond their middle years. Instead of building negative stress levels, involvement in a demanding, satisfying job has been shown to lessen our risk of the health problems that can be related to mid-life such as diabetes, ulcers, heart disease or depression. Negative stress appears to build if we are in an unsatisfying job coupled with a less than satisfactory home situation, especially if we feel powerless to change the situation. Challenges that we can meet, on the other hand, are an important ally in keeping us youthful.

Being positive

How many of us see life as a half-full or half-empty glass? If we instinctively interpret neutral events in a positive way, seeing opportunities to be grasped and positive changes to be made, we are far more likely to retain a youthful perspective on life. However, if we approach the same situation by responding fearfully, and anxiously feeling the threat of being unable to cope before we have even tried, we are very likely to age before we need to. After all, think of any tense people we know: the chances are that their worries and tensions are literally being etched on their face as time goes by, in the form of frown lines and wrinkles. Relaxed and positive people, on the other hand, get their fair share of age-related lines, but we often don't notice them in the same way because a relaxed face tends to be more mobile.

It has been suggested by Deepak Chopra, in *Ageless Ageing, Timeless Mind*, that in order to avoid a premature ageing experience we need to work on overturning any beliefs we hold that are supported by fear. So, instead of the negative belief that our bodies must inevitably decay day by day, we can replace this with the positive assertion that our bodies have the capacity to renew themselves minute by minute. Rather than regarding ourselves as machines that carry out certain tasks smoothly, but that can be subject to random malfunctions, we should instead concentrate on the potential our bodies have for self-regulation and maintaining positive health. Once we do this we can experience the joy of feeling that we are not at odds with our bodies. As a result, we are far more likely to be able to accept the direction in which we are moving.

The impact of stress on health and vitality

Is it possible to think ourselves healthy? Unlikely as it may sound to some of us, it is increasingly acknowledged that the state of our minds can have a profound effect on our physical experience of health. Two or three decades ago, if we took unexplained physical symptoms to our GPs, there was a good chance that they would be dismissed as being psychosomatic. Or, as it might be more commonly put, they were just 'all in the mind'. This wasn't generally of much help, since, apart from the option of psychiatric treatment, we wouldn't be given any further positive advice on how to make the necessary changes that might be needed to ease our psychosomatic problems.

Thank goodness we have all moved on, with the emerging field of psycho-neuro-immunology generating increasing attention and interest from the scientific establishment. Those who are working within this field have drawn attention to the way that negative reactions to stress can have a powerful impact on the body, which can reveal itself in a tendency to recurrent infections, and a reduced ability for the body to defend itself against serious illness.

As far back as the late 1970s, studies carried out at New York's Mount Sinai School of medicine demonstrated that emotionally stressful experiences such as grief and sadness could result in perceptible depression of our immune systems. Additional problems such as high blood pressure, digestive problems, and hardening of the arteries are also thought to be more likely to occur in those of us who are excessively over-loaded with negative stress.

In addition, work that has been carried out by Dr Carl Simonton and his wife Stephanie Matthews Simonton in the United States suggests that positive visualisation techniques may have an important role to play in helping cancer patients recover. Patients were encouraged to visualise their white cells fighting and overcoming the cancer, choosing imagery that was personal to them. The Simontons claimed that patients using this method on a regular basis lived on average twice as long as patients not using visualisation techniques.

There also appears to be a specific link between the need for stress reduction and enhancement of our experience of menopause. This is due to the way that we need a fundamentally healthy relationship between stress hormones and sex hormones if we are to experience optimum health and vitality at any age. It has been suggested that women who lead particularly stress-filled lives are likely to be at higher risk of experiencing distressing menopausal symptoms. This appears to be due to flagging adrenal gland reserves, since the adrenal glands provide some essential back-up to the ovaries as they begin to slow down oestrogen secretion.

It has been estimated that as much as 5 per cent of circulating sex hormones may be made up of adrenal gland secretions. As the ovaries secrete dwindling amounts of oestrogen, the adrenal glands can help pick up some of the slack by producing small amounts of oestrogen. In addition, they also double the production of male hormones that resemble testosterone (often referred to as androgens).

However, long-term stress can over-stress the adrenal glands, causing them to work at full stretch in order to produce stress hormones, including adrenaline. As a result, if we have exhausted adrenal glands we are unlikely to have the reserves we need in order to back up our hormone reserves at menopause and beyond.

The nature of stress

When we refer to stress as a single entity we are only considering part of the picture. Stress in itself is neutral, and a certain amount of positive stress is essential for us. Without it we would miss the necessary 'edge' that we need to help us perform in a focused and productive way. Positive stress gives us a slight flutter of butterflies in our stomach before we have to speak in public, or perform in an important interview. By being just stressed enough, we are likely to perform much better than we would if we felt too laid back.

Negative stress, on the other hand, tips us too far over the edge, holding us back from performing according to our maximum potential. This tends to happen when we have to cope on a regular basis with stress that we perceive as unmanageable. This often comes from confronting situations that we are powerless to solve to our advantage. After all, there is nothing quite so stressful as feeling we can't take action to change an unsatisfactory situation.

When we are experiencing negative stress on a daily basis we are unconsciously activating a stress response (often referred to as a 'flight or fight' mechanism). Although this is a perfectly appropriate and necessary reaction to a short-lived threat that demands physical action, it can be very damaging to our health if it becomes a regular feature of life.

This is due to the way that the fight or flight response activates the secretion of adrenaline in our bodies in addition to a range of other hormones that prepare us to deal with an emergency situation. The physical response involves blood being diverted from our digestive organs to our muscles in preparation for running, raises our heartbeat, and provides a general sense of heightened sensory awareness.

We can see straight away that this is extremely helpful if we need to sprint away from physical danger (which has the necessary effect of using up the adrenaline once it has done its job). On the other hand, if we react in this way whenever we are presented with an unexpectedly large phone bill, a difficult conversation with a family member, or an argument with our boss at work, we can see that we are soon going to land in deep trouble.

Apart from being one of the factors that can age us well before our time, persistent negative stress can cause a host of additional health problems including recurrent infections, constant fatigue, and cardiovascular disease. It can also have a significant impact on our experience of menopause. A revealing British study conducted in 1997 demonstrated how women who were stressed as a result of low educational status, combined with excessive workloads and poor psychological health, had a measurably more problematic and premature experience of menopause than other women.

Stress-busting techniques

Since negative stress is a fact of life for all of us at varying stages of our lives, it is vitally important that we discover how to deal with it. If we learn how to do this especially well we may even be empowered to turn it into positive stress, so that something negative can be turned around to work to our advantage.

The first thing which needs to be considered in any discussion of stress-proofing techniques is that some of us may be doing more harm than good by responding to ongoing stress with stress-defusing strategies that give only a temporary sense of relief. What is worse, these inappropriate responses to stress can make us feel even more negatively stressed in the long run, since they often involve using addictive substances such as alcohol, cigarettes, coffee, sugar or painkillers.

While each of the above will give us either the desired sense of relaxation (alcohol, cigarettes and painkillers) or a burst of energy (caffeinated drinks and anything made from refined sugar) in the short term, they only make us feel more stressed in the long term. This is due to the way that each of the items listed is addictive in nature, with the result that once the 'high' or 'low' has worn off, we are likely to feel that we need more of the substance in order to be able to cope.

So, in other words, if we have a cup of coffee and a chocolate bar in order to give us a boost of energy when we feel low, we will initially perk up and feel a sense of well-being and clear-headed-ness. However, the chances are that once the effect has worn off, we will rapidly begin to feel sluggish and drowsy once again. This leads to a growing need to reach for increasing quantities of caffeine and sugar to keep us going, with the result that we are very likely to end up feeling stressed, jittery, irritable, and have problems unwinding at night.

This can lead to a habit of taking a stiff gin or a couple of glasses of wine and a cigarette in the evenings in order to unwind and relax. This may often be topped off by taking a couple of painkillers or sleeping tablets in order to get a night's sleep. This, in turn, leads to feeling sluggish the next morning, so we get into a habit of starting off the day with strong coffee with a sugary cereal, and so the vicious circle goes on.

This approach is a little like the cosmetic response to signs of ageing described in the section above. In other words, we may gain the temporary illusion that we are solving our problems, but unless we tackle the more fundamental imbalance in our lifestyles, satisfying results are not going to be forthcoming. In fact, as we will see in the nutrition chapter, cigarettes, alcohol, caffeine and sugar have a definitely negative impact on our health when we are considering mid-life issues such as osteoporosis and heart disease.

Evaluating stress

Before we start considering stress-proofing our lives, we need to take a long, hard look at where the issues lie that are causing us most pressure. Once we do this, we are likely to become aware of how these issues that make us feel negatively stressed may be quite small in themselves, but it is their cumulative effect on us that is making us feel incapable of dealing effectively with them. Even more significantly, once we have identified the focus of our stresses we are in a position to take action, something which is in itself a major de-stressing tool.

Personal stress

- Unresolved tension in personal relationships.
- Adopting negative coping strategies.
- Lack of self-esteem.

Work-related stress

Common areas of stress may include any of the following:

- Problems with management of time.
- Difficulty in prioritising tasks.
- Putting up with a disorganised environment.
- Taking on unachievable goals.

Simple techniques for coping with personal stress

Unresolved tension in personal relationships

There is nothing quite so draining of personal sparkle and energy than putting up with relationships that are less than positive. Without realising it, we may be colluding in a negative solution by avoiding stating our needs clearly and firmly when we need to. This can affect a range of different relationships, including those we share with friends, partners, colleagues or family. If we constantly avoid important issues that need confronting in an effort to avoid stress in the short term, we may not realise that we are building bigger problems for ourselves in the future.

We should find by the time we reach mid-life that we have become sharply aware of our needs, and may be disinclined to put up with situations that do not have positive dimensions for us. After all, this can be one of the major benefits of getting older and having gathered experience. On the other hand, if our lives have become somewhat imbalanced over the years, we may find that we are involved in a series of relationships that are emotionally draining us, or making us feel that our needs are not being met.

If we find ourselves in this situation, we must take action, or we are likely to find that we pay a hefty price in terms of personal stress that can make our mid-life transition more problematic than it need be. Whatever action we take does not need to be drastic, but must be firm and considered, so that we are empowered to express our needs as clearly as possible.

It is essential not to mistake anger for assertiveness, since the latter involves clear-headedness – something that is certain to be lost once we have become angry. Once we have stated what we need as fairly as possible, this gives an opportunity to the other person to consider and understand our needs. It can also open up an important avenue of dialogue that can have a vital role to play in defusing unacknowledged stresses that may have built up over time.

The basic rule to remember is: if you are fuming over something, don't keep a stiff upper lip and keep it all inside. This is sure to lead to feeling drained, short-fused, and tense. Instead, bring it out into the open where it has a chance to be resolved.

Adopting negative coping strategies

Take a good, hard look at how you react to stressful times. Do you take refuge in stimulants (coffee and sugar) to keep going and sedatives (alcohol and prescription drugs) to unwind? Sadly, although this is a common reaction to negative stress, as we have seen in the section above, it brings its own problems with it. These often involve health problems that have a particular relevance to us as we approach and move through mid-life.

However, once these props are removed, we needn't feel as though that we have no choice but to be 'between a rock and a hard place'. On the contrary, once we develop fresh strategies that work in harmony with our bodies' own potential for stress-busting techniques, we are likely to feel delighted by the benefits that follow. Unlike the mood swings, jitteriness, or fuzzy-headedness that come with using the items listed above on a habitual basis, once we adopt a positive approach to stress-management we will begin to feel energised, focused, and enjoy the delight of feeling more in control of what may have seemed a previously unmanageable or out of control situation. In addition, we will also be freeing ourselves of the range of health risks associated with using potentially addictive substances

The strategies that we employ for turning negative coping strategies into positive ones may include freeing ourselves from poor eating and drinking habits (see Chapter 4 on 'Eating for the Long Run' for practical advice on how to set about this). Alternatively, if we feel that our main negative responses to stress are more bound up with an inability to relax and unwind, we would benefit from regularly practising one of the meditation or relaxation techniques outlined below.

Lack of self-esteem

It is difficult to improve the overall quality of our relationships if we don't first value and appreciate ourselves enough. In other words, if every time things go wrong we instinctively blame ourselves for it, we should stop for a moment and work out if this really is the case. The chances are that in many situations, we will probably have done the best that we could. On the other hand, if we have genuinely made a mistake that has contributed towards a difficult situation developing, we can turn this to our positive advantage by learning from it so that we don't keep on repeating the pattern.

Always blaming ourselves for things that go wrong is one of the greatest negative stress factors possible, since it is a fact of life that things will go awry from time to time. If every time this occurs we feel this provides us with evidence that we really are as incompetent, undesirable, unpopular, or unloved as we fear, this has the supremely negative effect of reinforcing our deepest insecurities. What is worse, this can set up a pattern which becomes self-fulfilling, since negative expectations can often result in negative outcomes.

The first step is to identify how negative assumptions about ourselves affect the way in which we interact with others, and how it may limit what we take on board. However, do bear in mind that what we are talking about here is different from a healthy and realistic awareness that there may be some tasks that we genuinely are not able to handle. In such a situation, saying no is perfectly appropriate, since taking on something that we know we aren't able to deal with effectively will only increase negative stress levels, and damage our confidence further.

On the other hand, if we are avoiding commitments that we rationally know we are perfectly equipped to handle effectively, but at the same time we lack sufficient confidence to take the plunge, we need to take action in order to free ourselves from the prison of self-doubt.

If patterns of flagging self-esteem are well established we would probably benefit from professional support and guidance in order to help us take the first vital steps. Cognitive therapy can be extremely helpful in assisting us to identify negative psychological conditioning that may have emerged during the formative years of childhood. Once these patterns are well established we continue to adopt them as adults, with the unfortunate result that they feel like second nature to us. A skilled therapist will be trained to help us identify and explore these patterns so that we begin to have a choice in how we respond to any potentially painful, difficult or stressful situation.

On the other hand, if we enjoy generally healthy levels of self-esteem but find that there are predictable times when we are subject to feelings of negativity about ourselves (for instance pre-menstrually), we may benefit greatly from alternative medical treatment which can encourage enhanced emotional equilibrium. Possible therapies to consider include homoeopathy, Western medical herbalism, or traditional Chinese medicine.

Simple techniques for coping with work-related stress

Problems with time management

In order to manage stress levels as effectively as possible we need to pace ourselves at work and at home at a level that suits us as individuals. Nothing is likely to make us feel as stressed out, and appear as tense and edgy, as feeling that we just don't have enough time to do all that we need to accomplish in an effective way. For many of us, perpetually feeling tense etches itself on our faces and necks where signs of stress are first likely to show, making us look old before our time. In addition, feeling under this degree of pressure also results in persistent problems with tension head-aches, migraines, back pain, and a host of digestive problems that can span the range from mild indigestion to full-blown symptoms of irritable bowel syndrome.

However, we needn't put up with feeling like a hamster on an exercise wheel who runs all day in order to keep still; all it takes to break the cycle is a considered look at how we are structuring our day. As with so many problems of this kind, acknowledging that we have a problem is our first important step towards finding a solution.

If we find that problems start at the beginning of the day because we have a tendency to leave everything to the last minute, it really is worth making a point of getting up an extra half hour before we need to. This will reduce the tendency to dash around in a panic, with the desirable result that things will tend to go much more smoothly. The same applies to travelling to work: if we know that it takes at least half an hour, it helps enormously to give ourselves an extra fifteen minutes or so, so that we can accommodate a small delay without tearing our hair out in desperation.

During the day, make a point of prioritising known tasks (see below for advice on how this can be effectively done), trying not to get unduly distracted by unimportant side issues. Also build in small gaps so that there isn't a sense of moving without respite from one task to another – a sure-fire way of getting burnt out.

Also make a definite point of structuring life at home so that some relaxation time is available on a daily basis. Without this essential support we are less likely to be productive and focused when we need to be. Relaxation time doesn't need to take up hours, it can be anything from twenty to thirty minutes or an hour. We should choose whatever suits us as individuals, and makes us feel most relaxed and refreshed. According to our personalities this could be anything from enjoying a formal relaxation technique, to taking a walk in the fresh air, doing an exercise class, listening to music, reading a favourite novel, or having a leisurely bath with scented oils and candlelight.

Above all else, effective management of time works best when we make a point of being realistic about what we can actually achieve. Always avoid falling into the trap of trying to do what is physically impossible; there is nothing quite as frustrating or exhausting as trying to achieve the impossible.

Prioritising tasks

Feeling snowed under by a mountain of professional or domestic commitments is one of the most draining problems we can encounter. However, it is enormously important to realise that we can use simple techniques that can diminish the scale of the problem at a single stroke. Once we do this, what seemed to be a problem of insurmountable proportions shrinks to a much more manageable size. This is likely to have the instant effect of making us feel relieved and much less stressed.

The simplest way of establishing pressing priorities is to make a list of what must be done. Simple as it sounds, this basic technique helps us organise and clarify our thoughts, which prevents us from feeling as though we are so overwhelmed that we don't know how or where to start. It is vitally important to move beyond this negative state of mind, since feeling bogged down by small details will cause us to feel indecisive, confused, and more stressed out than ever. As a result, we are in less of a position to act with clarity, so that nothing positive gets done and we will be left feeling increasingly tense and guilty.

Once we focus on writing down the activities we need to tackle, the physical act of writing distances us slightly from the subject we are writing about, with the natural consequence that tasks requiring obvious priority tend to stand out. Making lists also brings with it the important benefit of focusing the mind, empowering us to think with more clarity about what we need to do.

It may sound obvious, but it helps greatly if we organise lists in terms of priority. So tasks that demand immediate attention should occupy positions at the top of the list, while less pressing jobs should be included further down. It also helps if we have a way of coding tasks that need to be tackled straight away, or those that can be delayed for a while without causing any problems or complications.

Don't waste time spending important mental energy on worrying about jobs that don't really need to be tackled at all, or that can be delegated to someone else. Strike them off the list, or make a note to hand them over to someone else straight away – you will be surprised to discover how powerful a stress-reduction technique it can be to see a list shrinking in this way.

Putting up with a disorganised environment

If we feel stressed to the hilt, it can be very helpful to stop for a moment and take a quick glance at our surroundings. This can be extremely illuminating since, for many of us, our external environmental often reflects the state of mind that we are in. When we feel under excessive pressure, mentally disorganised, and incapable of dealing with the sheer scale of what we have to do, this mental state is often reinforced by our being surrounded by a jumble of disorganised books and papers without being consciously aware of it.

Thankfully, we can do a great deal to relieve ourselves of emotional and mental pressure by tackling and organising our professional and domestic surroundings. On a purely practical level, work of any kind is so much easier and more productive if we can find the material we need quickly and with ease. On the other hand, just think of the frustration and waste of time that inevitably occur when, working under pressure, we spend precious time searching through endless heaps of paper.

It does help to bear in mind, as with everything else that we have discussed in this book, that what we are searching for here is an optimum sense of balance and equilibrium. In other words, when all is well, we shouldn't find that we become so preoccupied with neatness and organisation that our behaviour becomes close to obsessional. If we drift into this undesirable frame of mind, it can be identified when the desire to control our external environment takes over from every other consideration. Sadly, this is a totally negative situation to be in, since putting so much energy into fruitlessly trying to control things around us makes us too tense and exhausted to live life creatively.

However, once a healthy balance between these two extremes has been struck, keeping our immediate environment in an ordered state becomes a tool that supports us in working to our maximum potential. As a direct consequence, it can be immensely helpful in defusing negative stress and preventing us from being at the mercy of feeling passive and ineffective.

Taking on unachievable goals

If we are to feel less stressed we always need to be careful that we work within stimulating and realistic boundaries for ourselves. There is nothing quite so sure to lead us to a state of burn-out as taking on commitments that we can't possibly fulfil to the best of our ability. However tempting it may be to believe that we are superwomen, if we are constantly overburdening ourselves with unrealistic commitments, the unfortunate common result is a diminishing sense of self-esteem and self-confidence.

What we are striving for once again is a healthy balance of stress that makes us feel we are being stretched, so that we continue to grow and develop. In order to make the most of these opportunities, we must feel able to tackle whatever is at hand to the best of our ability. One of the major allies we have at our disposal in achieving this is the important skill of being able to say no to any tasks we genuinely consider inappropriate for us to tackle. This need not be exploited as an opportunity to shy away from realistic demands, but can be a valuable way of ridding ourselves of unrealistic pressures that may be causing us disproportionate stress.

Women are well known as having greater skills than men in being able to juggle a number of tasks at once. On the other hand, this gift can leave us open to the tendency to try to do an unrealistic amount within a professional as well as a domestic context, and when we fail (as we will inevitably do if the demands are unreasonable), we may blame ourselves for not being competent or successful enough.

It can be immensely helpful as a stress-management technique to regularly evaluate our workloads in order to check that they have remained within realistic boundaries. Doing this on a fairly regular basis can combat the tendency for commitments to grow insidiously without our consciously realising it. If we leave it for too long, things may have reached near breaking point before our alarm bells begin to ring.

Delegating tasks can also be a magnificent way of keeping our professional or domestic demands within healthy boundaries. It is also one of the most positive tools of stress management that we can have at our disposal. We are most likely to delegate efficiently if we are good at prioritising tasks as outlined above. By being able to see clearly which tasks are essential and which tasks are less pressing, we are also going to have a good idea of those jobs that must be done by us, and those that can be passed on to others to do for us. Of course, this applies as much to domestic commitments as it does to professional pressures.

On a purely psychological level, once we develop the ability to ask for help, we are well on the way to feeling immensely liberated as well as dealing much more efficiently with the demands that present themselves to us. It can also come as a surprise and a huge relief to discover that we are not as indispensable as we may once have thought. Of course, if we are used to feeling indispensable we are likely to find that it is difficult to take the first step in handing over and letting go of certain tasks. However, although this can be painful at first, once we become effective delegators we may be amazed to discover how this can substantially reduce our stress level virtually overnight.

General stress-proofing techniques: the relaxation response

It often used to be said that anybody could relax, the general impression being given that this was something everybody could instinctively just tap into if they set their minds to it. While this may be true to a certain extent, it is now much more readily accepted that relaxation often requires more specific skills in order to help those who aren't 'naturals' at relaxing to 'switch off'. The irony, of course, is that these latter are very often the people who are most in need of learning how to induce what has been termed the relaxation response.

Benefits of learning how to relax are wide-ranging and may include greater clarity of thought, improved energy levels, sounder sleep, and fewer physical aches and pains or headaches that are related to muscle tension. Since relaxation techniques are known to be our first line of defence in any effective stress-reduction plan, they also appear to have beneficial effects on our immune-system performance, in addition to having a balancing effect on hormonal secretions when they are practised on a regular basis.

As we can imagine, this has a particular relevance for us at menopause, since it is acknowledged that the specific symptoms that can arise at this time can be made worse or eased by how well we deal with stress. Hot flushes, night sweats, anxious episodes, persistent fatigue and poor sleep pattern are all likely to be made more severe and troublesome by an excessively stressful lifestyle. These symptoms, in turn, can make us feel even more uptight, and so the vicious circle can go on. Setting aside time to relax each day can give us the tool that we need to break this negative pattern, empowering us to recharge and re-balance our systems.

Basic background to relaxation

Correct breathing
Correct breathing is an invaluable aid to achieving a calm and relaxed state. Although we breathe in and out countless times during the day, the way in which we do this as a general rule is classed as being involuntary. In other words, it takes place as an unconscious reflex, with our attention only being likely to be drawn to it if we feel a sense of irregularity or uncharacteristic uneasiness in our breathing pattern. On the other hand, if we want to induce a sense of mental and physical relaxation, we need to become aware of how to breathe from the diaphragm (the sheet of muscle that extends across the base of the rib cage).

When we first learn how to breathe to induce a relaxed state, it helps to lie on the floor with our knees bent, with feet about a foot or so apart. Alternatively, we can choose to sit in a straight-backed chair with feet resting firmly on the floor. In order to establish that we are breathing diaphragmatically we need to rest one hand lightly on the area just above the navel. As we take a deep breath in we should feel our hand rise gently as our lungs fill fully with air, making sure that we keep our shoulders down and relaxed. As we fully breathe out, we should feel our hands sinking back to their original position as our bellies contract and we expel air from the base of our lungs to the top.

If any dizziness or sense of disorientation occurs, take a few natural breaths and begin diaphragmatic breathing once again when you feel ready. Above all, listen to what your body is telling you and never force the breaths. Always let them happen at their own pace and rhythm.

Combining pleasurable activities

Experiment with combining pleasurable activities that promote feelings of increased well-being and relaxation. So, we may maximise the soothing effects of a warm, leisurely bath by adding a few drops of relaxing essential oils, lighting candles which give a softer glow than electric lights, and listening to a favourite piece of music.

A healthy sleep pattern

Make a point of maintaining a healthy pattern of good quality, restful sleep in order to keep tension and stress at bay. There is no hard and fast rule that tells us what the optimum amount of sleep is for everyone, since each of us is likely to have slightly different requirements. We should follow our instincts and adopt a sleep pattern that feels as though it is meeting our requirements in duration and depth of sleep. When these are being appropriately met, we should feel refreshed on waking, energised through the day, and relaxed enough at night to fall asleep readily and effortlessly.

Do remember that apart from defusing stress, a healthy, regular sleep pattern also provides us with a vital anti-ageing tool. This is due to the way that all of our major organs go into a restful mode during sleep, while our immune systems have a chance to recharge themselves, thus making them more capable of fighting the effects of rampaging free radicals in our bodies. In addition, we secrete growth hormone in our sleep which enables our bodies to renew and repair themselves. It has been suggested that every tissue in our bodies appear to be renewed and regenerated at a faster rate during sound sleep than in our waking hours.

Aerobic exercise

Regular, aerobic exercise also provides an excellent context within which we can enjoy the benefits of relaxation. Aerobic activities such as brisk walking and cycling play an important positive role in helping us burn off the excess adrenaline that is produced when we have a sedentary, stressful occupation that doesn't give us the chance to release built-up tension through physical activity when we need to.

Relaxation techniques

Autogenic training

This is a formal relaxation technique that we can learn in order to gain control over feelings of random panic and anxiety. Once we become familiar with the skills of autogenic training we can use them at will in order to induce a deep state of relaxation. Even functions of the body that are usually not considered to be under our conscious control (such as pulse or heart rate) are thought to benefit from the state of profound relaxation that can be induced by autogenic training.

If we want to learn how to use this technique effectively, it is best first to seek training from a qualified practitioner, rather than trying to learn the basic skills by ourselves. The technique involves mastering half a dozen mental exercises which involve the suggestion that certain, very specific sensations are being experienced such as warmth, heaviness or calmness in specified parts of the body. However, we do need guidance and training from a skilled practitioner to start with, because certain psychological reactions may occur in response to autogenic training. If this should happen, it helps enormously if the assessment of an experienced practitioner is available to evaluate these reactions.

Once we are skilled and familiar with practising autogenic training, we can use it to trigger a deeply relaxed state whenever we need to do so. It helps to bear in mind that this is a very practical system of relaxation that can be used at any time, anywhere. As a result, we can make the most of the benefits of a swiftly induced state of relaxation with the minimum amount of fuss and bother. It helps if the technique is practised on a regular basis, since this helps us develop the sharp sense of subjective observation that comes as we become familiar with the different sensations of deep relaxation.

Meditation

Daily practice of meditation can play an important role in helping us feel a sense of increased calmness and tranquillity on a mental, emotional and physical level. Once we feel more laid back and generally relaxed, we should find that we reap the additional benefit of improved levels of concentration and increased clarity of thought. This can be an invaluable asset at stressful times when we may feel stretched to our mental and emotional limit. If we also bear in mind that forgetfulness and poor concentration are very common symptoms that cause a great deal of distress at menopause, the potential benefits that meditation can bring are especially valuable and relevant.

We can induce a meditative state by sitting in a pleasantly warm, peaceful environment. Choose a chair which has a high, straight back in order to give the best chance for your spine to be supported in maximum alignment. As you sit in as relaxed a posture as possible, consciously free your mind of busy, distracting thoughts. This process will be aided by focusing on an image – either something placed in front of you, or a purely mentally generated image. Common images that are used to induce a meditative state include a flower or a candle.

On the other hand, if you respond more strongly to sound than a visual image, it may feel more appropriate to close your eyes and repeat a sound to yourself over and over again. This needn't be anything more complicated than repeating the word 'one', as you observe and regulate your breathing pattern. It is likely that distracting thoughts will periodically float into your mind. Irritating as this can be, don't panic or become discouraged, but mentally put them to one side and focus once again on your chosen sound or image.

Step-by-step relaxation

The following is a simple relaxation exercise that can be done each day in order to reduce tension, ease muscular aches and pains, and clear the mind.

- Before starting to relax, make sure that you are dressed in clothes that are warm, loose, and extremely comfortable.
- The temperature of the room is also very important, since entering a state of deep relaxation causes the body temperature to drop significantly. If we begin to feel uncomfortably cold, this can be distracting and obstruct our feeling fully mentally and physically relaxed.
- Lie on the floor with knees bent and feet a hip width apart. Rest one hand on your belly so that you can check that you are breathing from your diaphragm, rather than from your upper chest. See advice given above on correct breathing techniques in order to learn how to breathe for maximum relaxation.
- Let your breathing follow its own comfortable pace rather than forcing the breath. Ideally all you need to do is observe what is happening.
- Once diaphragmatic breathing is established, let your legs relax to the floor so that your whole leg is in contact with the surface on which you are lying. Your arms should also rest against the floor with the hands relaxed and loose; ideally the palms should be facing upwards with the fingers gently curled and open.
- Concentrate initially on the muscles of your face and head. Starting at the crown of your head, visualise letting go of the tension in the muscles of your scalp. Move down your forehead

and face in the same way, taking note of any tightness you encounter on your way, and consciously releasing it.

- As the facial and neck muscles relax, you should feel a sense of softness enter your eyes, nose, cheeks, lips, jaw and throat. Your lips may naturally part a little as a result of general relaxation of the face and jaw. Don't try to fight this, since it is a positive sign which indicates that you are entering a state of relaxation.

- Repeat the same process for each area of your body in turn, moving in downward sequence from your neck to the shoulders, upper arms, lower arms, hands, chest, abdomen, buttocks, upper thighs, knees, calves, ankles, feet and toes. During this process you are likely to become aware of localised areas that are obviously tense and tight. These are the areas that must have extra time spent on them, until they begin to feel fully relaxed and loosened.

- Once this process is fully under way you should feel distinctly relaxed and comfortable. It is a common sensation to feel as though our bodies have become much heavier when we fully relax, almost as though they are sinking through the floor. Some of us, on the other hand, may experience the reverse sensation and feel as though we are floating slightly above the surface on which we are lying.

- Once you are completely relaxed, you should bring your attention back to your breathing pattern. You should find that it has naturally slowed down and regulated itself to a natural, steady, relaxed rhythm.

- As you are focusing on your breathing you should begin to visualise a bright light filling your body with positive mental and physical energy as you breathe in, while imagining toxic waste and traces of negativity leaving your body as you breathe out. Choose whatever colours or images feel appropriate or attractive, and change them as often as feels appropriate.

- Stay in this relaxed state for as long as feels appropriate, or for as long as practical demands allow. Always allow enough time to emerge from this experience of deep relaxation, since it is important this shouldn't be rushed if you are to hold on to the benefits of the exercise.

- Once you are ready, begin by bringing your attention slowly back to your surroundings. Move your head, hands and feet slowly in turn, building up from small movements to gentle flexings and stretchings. Finally give one whole body stretch and open your eyes.
- Slowly roll on to one side, and spend a little time sitting up before standing. This is done in order to avoid the dizziness or disorientation that can result from getting up too abruptly.

Once we have built a regular relaxation slot into our daily routine, we are likely to be amazed at the benefits that follow. Apart from the positive mental, emotional and physical aspects to relaxation and meditation already mentioned, there is a more basic advantage that should not be overlooked. By giving ourselves the necessary space and time within which to relax, we are acknowledging our needs as the first priority. For many of us this is likely to feel unusually difficult at first, since many women will instinctively care for others before spending valuable time on nurturing themselves.

However, once we learn how to give ourselves the necessary space that we need in order to recharge and renew our emotional batteries, we are far more likely to feel we have the vital mental, emotional and physical balance that we need to meet our own and others' needs most effectively. Once we make relaxation a basic part of our lives, within a short time we are likely to wonder how on earth we managed without it!

Now we have considered stress reduction as the fundamental tool we have at our disposal in preparing for menopause, it's time to move on to the two other basic areas of essential lifestyle support: nutrition and exercise. A detailed discussion of the importance of both is given in the next two chapters.

4

Eating for the Long Run

Most of us will be very aware by now of the importance of sound nutrition and the direct effect it has on the overall quality of health that we enjoy. After all, we are bombarded by the latest advice on healthy eating from articles in newspapers, magazines, and the Internet, while most television slots that deal with health issues will always give high priority to discussions about healthy and un-healthy eating. We are probably more concerned than we have ever been about the merits of low-fat and low-sugar eating plans, while the debate about organic produce is extremely hot news just now.

The reason why this is so is really very straightforward, since many of us have come to realise that we literally are what we eat. In other words, whatever foods and drinks we choose to consume on a regular basis will form the basic building blocks from which our bodies will be able to repair and renew themselves, as well as determining how much energy and vitality we enjoy.

In the recent past there was a tendency to assume that there was a 'quick fix' for most health problems. So, if we were constantly developing one infection after another, why worry, since there were antibiotics on hand to knock the infection out? The same could be said of the tendency to rely on antacids and laxatives as a way of keeping digestive problems at bay, rather than attending to matters in our diets or lifestyle that might be leading to the problems in the first place. More significantly, many of us may have learnt too late about the serious drawbacks associated with the 'magic bullet' approach to treating emotional problems such as anxiety with tranquillisers. Even now, there are growing concerns about the negative aspects of relying on more modern antidepressants such as Prozac.

As a direct result of an awareness that excessive dependence on conventional drugs to solve our health problems will too frequently leave us disappointed, many of us have come to take a more holistic view on looking after our health and sense of well-being. This broader, more supportive approach may be regarded as a form of preventive medicine, with a great deal of the emphasis being put on ways we can improve our general health. One of the most fundamental ways of doing this is through sound nutrition, and nowhere is this of greater importance than when we are approaching and moving beyond the menopause.

Why what we eat is of central importance as we move through menopause

Given what has already been said, the limitations of a drug-based approach in easing us through the transitional phase of menopause are obvious. Concerns about increased risk of breast cancer and heart disease apart (see Chapter 6, 'The Pros and Cons of Hormone Replacement Therapy', for a general discussion of these problems), there are additional issues connected with taking HRT that are related to the 'quick-fix' argument outlined above. After all, very few of us who consult our GPs are likely to be given the detailed essential information we need to give ourselves maximum protection against heart disease and osteoporosis by making necessary adjustments to our lifestyles. These changes include important dietary measures and taking the idea of physical fitness very seriously.

Although conventional doctors may be aware of some of these issues, there is often a tendency to consider the major menopausal problems such as osteoporosis as being dealt with by taking HRT, leaving lifestyle issues as helpful, but essentially subsidiary or optional extras. As a result, many of us may pin all of our hopes on HRT to solve our problems at menopause without being aware of the essential changes we can make to support our bodies through this vitally important transition.

It has been suggested by nutritional therapists such as Marilyn Glenville, or medical herbalists such as Kitty Campion, that adopting a sound and well-informed approach to nutrition, and a generally health-promoting lifestyle during the years leading up to and beyond the menopause may render more drastic measures such as hormone replacement therapy unnecessary. It is certainly undeniable that realistically evaluating the quality of our daily eating habits should be one of the first things that we do if we are looking to improve the overall quality of our health in our middle years and beyond. By taking basic nutritional action at as early a stage as possible we can lessen our risk of developing a range of degenerative chronic conditions such as arthritis, while guarding against unnecessary mood swings and chronic fatigue.

If we have more specific goals in mind, such as protecting ourselves against osteoporosis and heart disease, our nutritional status assumes an even greater significance, since both these conditions have been shown to be aggravated or improved by the quality of the food we eat, in addition to general aspects of our lifestyle, such as the way in which we handle stress and the amount of exercise that we take.

Although in an ideal world whatever eating plan we adopt should always meet our individual needs and requirements as closely as possible, there are very general hints that we should try to follow if we want to have the maximum chance of protecting our overall health at menopause. Once we have these firmly in place, we can go on to explore in greater depth more specific nutritional advice that can help us deal with common menopausal problems.

Do remember that what we are ideally looking at from this point onwards is a fresh approach to our patterns of eating that we can continue for the rest of our lives if we want to have the chance of enjoying maximum health and vitality. In other words, this is a long-term objective which is the complete opposite of the 'quick-fix' approach. As we have already seen, however attractive the latter may be when we want a fast solution, the inevitable drawback is that problems often return with irritating regularity if we haven't attended to underlying contributing problems in our lifestyles.

The basic foundation of sound nutrition at menopause

Balancing blood sugar levels

Stable blood sugar levels are important at any stage of life if we are avoid the symptoms of low blood sugar or hypoglycaemia (these include fatigue, dizziness, lack of concentration, and mood swings). However, the issue of keeping blood sugar levels at their optimum level becomes of particular relevance and importance as we approach and move through menopause. If our blood sugar levels are kept at a stable 'cruising level' we are able to make maximum use of the female hormones that are produced by our bodies. As a result, we should find that this helps to discourage problems developing with common menopausal symptoms such as hot flushes.

The two main factors that influence our blood sugar levels are the quality of the food that has been eaten, and the length of the gap between each meal. Eating too much refined food (anything that is made from white sugar and white flour), and too many junk foods such as fizzy drinks, chocolate and sweets will cause a rapid rise in blood sugar, because they are digested so rapidly. Stimulants such as tea, coffee and alcohol have a similar effect on the body, causing the bloodstream to be swiftly flooded with sugar. Once this happens, the common response of the body is to bring down blood sugar levels as quickly as possible through secreting insulin from the pancreas, with the result that we are likely to feel a resulting dip in energy and concentration as this occurs. This often leads us to reach for more sweets, coffee or caffeinated fizzy drinks in order to get another energy high. This sets off a vicious cycle of energy highs and lows that leave us with a trigger-happy, and eventually exhausted pancreas.

On the other hand, if we leave too long between meals (more

than three hours or so in women) we can experience persistently low blood sugar levels. If we go for a quick snack such as a coffee and a cake, we are likely to get a sugar 'rush' that results in the same negative blood sugar cycle outlined above. More significantly, low blood sugar stimulates secretion of the stress hormone adrenalin from the adrenal glands. Adrenalin has a major impact on our whole system by preparing our bodies for a 'fight or flight' response. This involves speeding up our heart rates, increasing blood pressure, slowing down digestion, and freeing up emergency stores of sugar into our blood streams. While these reactions are all appropriate when we need to prepare our bodies to face a physical threat that requires physical action, they rapidly become inappropriate if they are occurring several times a day in response to ongoing psychological stress or an inadequate or inappropriate diet. This is a particularly relevant issue when we reach menopause and beyond, since our adrenal glands can supply us with additional oestrogen as well as secreting a natural hormone called DHEA that may have potent anti-ageing properties.

Simple tips for balancing blood sugar

- Make sure that plenty of helpings of complex carbohydrates are included in your daily diet, since these have an important role to play in stabilising blood sugar, unlike refined carbohydrates which have the opposite effect. Complex carbohydrates (these include items made from whole-wheat flour such as bread and pasta, brown rice, and starchy vegetables such as potatoes eaten with their skins intact) have the desirable effect of giving us a slow, sustained energy release. Enjoying frequent snacks of complex carbohydrates every two or three hours can help deal with cravings for junk, quick, 'energy-fix' foods, while also keeping feelings of anxiety at bay that may be sparked off by erratic blood sugar levels.
- Avoid refined (white) sugar whenever possible. Take care to examine ingredients used in convenience foods, since significant amounts of refined sugar are included in a surprising range of savoury items such as baked beans, mayonnaise, salad creams,

tomato ketchup, chutneys and pickles. Although, generally speaking, fruit sugar is less of a problem in destabilising blood sugar when it is eaten as a piece of fruit, if it is drunk in the form of juice it can cause a rapid rise in blood sugar because of the absence of fibre to slow down the process of absorption. Apart from its negative effect on blood sugar levels, refined sugar has the added drawback that all of its fibre, vitamins, minerals and trace elements have been removed during the refining process. Since our bodies use up existing vitamins and minerals during the process of digesting sweet items, refined sugar may be regarded as being nutritionally 'empty'.

- Cut down drastically, or eliminate stimulant foods and drinks altogether. These include any caffeinated drinks such as coffee, tea, chocolate or fizzy colas (these have a double disadvantage of including a hefty amount of refined sugar in addition to caffeine). Also watch out for painkillers that include caffeine as an ingredient to counteract the drowsiness of codeine. These can contribute to rebound headaches as well as unstable blood sugar levels. There appear to be very strong links between the use of stimulants and an erratic rise and fall of blood sugar levels, as well as an increased possibility of more frequent and severe hot flushes due to increased dilation (expansion) of blood vessels. Spicy foods should also be avoided for the same reason because of their tendency to encourage the body to sweat in order to cool itself down.

Reducing red meat and dairy products

Many of us by now will be aware of the problems connected with eating red meat due its saturated fat content which has been linked to an increased risk of developing heart and circulatory disease. We may also know that frequent consumption of red meat can increase the possibility of developing bowel cancer. This is due to the way that red meat moves so slowly through the digestive tract (unlike fruit, vegetables, pulses or fish) that there is a tendency for it to putrefy in the gut. Of course, red meat is also controversial because of the debate about BSE, but there are additional issues connected to consumption of red meat that are of special relevance to us as we approach menopause. This involves concern about the way in which hormone supplementation is used in the farming of animals in order to increase weight gain and improve meat quality. Red meats such as beef, pork, or game may leave us open to increased risk of oestrogen imbalance (oestrogen supplementation may be used to improve the quality of the meat), while also leaving us more vulnerable to the development of osteoporosis because of their high phosphate content. The latter is also a particular problem with preserved meats such as bacon and ham, which should be avoided wherever possible for the same reason. The use of growth hormones in meat production is also questionable, since apart from encouraging problems with unstable blood sugar levels and blood pressure irregularities, growth hormones may also be implicated in increased risk of breast cancer. If cutting out red meat is not an option, make a point of cutting down substantially on the amount eaten, and of buying organic produce.

Dairy foods may be eaten in moderation, but it should be borne in mind that cows' milk and products made from cows' milk may be difficult to digest for many of us. As a result, a diet which contains large quantities of dairy foods may have the undesirable effect of blocking vital nutrients from being used as they need to be by the body. Dairy foods can also aggravate symptoms of fatigue, persistent catarrh, and a tendency to recurring chesty coughs because of increased mucus production. Many dairy foods such as full-fat cheeses also have the drawback of being high in saturated fat, which is of particular relevance if we are concerned about the increased risk of heart disease after the menopause. It also helps to remember that while dairy foods are rich in calcium, these are not the only source for this essential mineral. Important non-dairy sources include soya beans, sesame seeds, oily fish that are eaten with their bones (salmon and sardines), and green leafy vegetables.

Increasing the amount of fibre eaten on a daily basis

This has an important dual effect of contributing to increased stability of blood sugar levels while also guarding against persistent problems with constipation. Many of us may find that the latter can be an annoying problem that comes with menopause, leading to associated irritating symptoms of bloating, and excess wind which we understandably feel we could well do without. The following are simple and painless ways of increasing our daily fibre intake:

- Make a habit of always choosing whole grain versions of bread, pasta and rice in preference to the refined varieties which have been largely stripped of their fibre content.
- Avoid foods that contain a mixture of unhealthy fats (saturated and hydrogenated), refined flour and refined sugar. This combination is generally most likely to be found in convenience foods, cakes, biscuits, and commercially produced puddings.
- Include at least five portions of raw, or lightly steamed fresh vegetables and fruit each day.
- Above all, avoid the trap of thinking that a quick-fix solution to too little fibre being included in the diet can be solved by sprinkling bran on food. Always bear in mind that bran is actually a refined product with few of the positive qualities that we obtain from wholegrain foods. In addition, it binds to certain minerals, preventing their absorption by the body. As a result, regular use of bran can result in poor absorption of iron, zinc and magnesium.

Reducing salt intake

Many of us will already be aware of the dangers of taking too much salt in connection with problems of high blood pressure and increased risk of heart disease and strokes. However, it has also been suggested that an excess of salt in the diet may leave us more vulnerable to the development of osteoporosis. This is thought to be connected to increased secretion of calcium in proportion to the salt that is ingested. What we should be aiming for is an optimum balance in our bodies between sodium and potassium, a balance that becomes impossible if we take large quantities of salt each day. Convenience foods are generally major sources of added salt in the form of monosodium glutamate, sodium bicarbonate, sodium benzoate and sodium citrate. Additional foods that contain surprising amounts of added salt include breakfast cereals, evaporated milk, hard cheeses, and even medicines such as antacids that contain sodium bicarbonate. The following are basic suggestions of how to rectify a sodium/potassium imbalance:

- Cut down on items that encourage a deficiency of potassium. These include coffee, sugar, alcohol, diuretics and laxatives.
- Drastically reduce or eliminate from the diet foods that are a generous source of sodium. It has been estimated that we need no more than 4 g on a daily basis in order to maintain optimum fluid balance. However, many of us take up to 20 g a day on a regular basis by adding salt to our food, and indirectly through 'hidden' salt in some of the foods mentioned above. Common symptoms that suggest we are taking an excess of salt include fluid retention, fatigue, and poor ability to fight infection.
- Include extra foods every day in the diet that are a good source of potassium, such as fresh fruit and vegetables.

Reducing intake of alcohol and other addictive drinks

Many of us may instinctively find that as we get older we just can't keep the pace and tolerate alcohol in the way we used to. Suddenly, a couple of glasses of wine will have the same effect that twice that quantity or more used to have a decade ago. The reason for this is that our bodies have less of a capacity for flushing toxins out of the tissues when we are forty than they did when we were twenty. As a result of this ongoing process, we are sure to discover that we have less of a capacity for tolerating alcohol, nicotine, or even coffee and tea than we did when we were younger. On the other hand, if we keep our daily intake well within, and ideally significantly beneath recommended limits (fourteen units of alcohol a week and a maximum of one cup of coffee a day) we are still likely to enjoy the odd glass of wine or cup of coffee, without having to feel toxic as payment for our pleasure.

We need to take particular care with how we handle addictive substances as we move closer to menopause, since alcohol, cigarettes, tea and coffee have particular drawbacks associated with them with regard to our overall health and well-being at this time. Apart from generally feeling unwell, headachy and sluggish if we over-indulge in alcohol, cigarettes or coffee, we are also substantially increasing our risk of osteoporosis if we consume significant quantities of any of these on a regular basis.

To be honest, we really should be aiming to give up smoking altogether if we want to enjoy the best chance of optimum health and vitality at menopause. When we smoke we significantly increase our risk of heart and circulatory disease (smokers run a 70 per cent increased risk of developing a heart attack) as well as cancer of the lungs, while at the same time compromising our bone density (it has been suggested that smoking can decrease bone mass by anything up to 25 per cent). In addition, smoking has powerful ageing effects on our skin due to its disastrous effect on collagen, plus the way in which it depletes our bodies of essential nutrients such as vitamin C, bioflavinoids and zinc. If we add in the increased risk that smokers run of developing debilitating chronic chest problems such as bronchitis and emphysema, is it really worth keeping up the habit?

Alcohol brings a related series of problems with it when taken too frequently or in excessive quantities. These include a tendency to unstable blood sugar levels and an increased risk of liver damage. It also prevents us from making maximum use of the nutrients that we ingest by blocking the absorption of essential fatty acids and zinc, as well as leaving us more vulnerable to developing osteoporosis. However, unlike smoking which has absolutely no benefit associated to it, there are some positive aspects to extremely moderate consumption of alcohol, so we need not feel that a drop of alcohol should never pass our lips again. The key lies in making sure that this doesn't cross over sensible boundaries where it becomes a health hazard. A glass of good quality red wine a day appears to have a protective effect on our circulatory systems as well as providing us with some nutrients such as vitamins A and B complex. In addition, a small quantity of wine stimulates the appetite by getting digestive juices flowing, which creates favourable conditions for easy digestion. However, it is still a good idea to have a regular alcohol-free period when our livers are given a chance to rest and regenerate themselves. During these phases, we needn't feel deprived since we can enjoy the increasing range of herb-based soft drinks available on the market that are also free of large quantities of refined sugar or artificial sweeteners.

Coffee also needs to be treated with a degree of caution and respect since it has particular problems associated with it if we are concerned about our overall health at menopause. Many of us will probably already know that there are links between high coffee intake and stress-related symptoms such as headaches, jitteriness, indigestion and irritability. However, there are specific menopausal problems that can be significantly aggravated by regular coffee consumption such as poor sleep quality, hot flushes, anxiety, depression and fatigue. In addition, drinking anything between one and two cups of strong coffee a day has been linked with a significantly increased risk of osteoporosis. Since regular coffee drinking can also aggravate high blood pressure, it could also be argued that we would be taking a positive step in looking after our hearts and circulatory systems if we drastically cut down our coffee drinking. Coffee also has a powerful diuretic effect which encourages the leaching of essential nutrients from our bodies, as well as leaving us more susceptible to develop painful, lumpy breasts.

Although tea has less caffeine per cup than coffee, it can lead to similar problems by contributing to the malabsorption of calcium, zinc, iron and magnesium. We also need to treat chocolate, cocoa and fizzy cola-type drinks with as much care as coffee, since they include the addictive properties of caffeine and sugar, as well as the problems associated with phosphorus in the case of cola-type, sweet, fizzy drinks (these can aggravate a tendency to osteoporosis).

When we set about cutting out addictive drinks it helps to know that it's generally best to find palatable substitutes that we can introduce first, so that we don't start to feel deprived and resentful. If we need to drastically cut down a high coffee intake, it's best not to try this overnight, in order to avoid the miseries of caffeine withdrawal. The latter can involve anything from a sickening headache, to feeling nauseated, jittery and bad-tempered. Try instead to reduce the number of cups of coffee you drink slowly and steadily by substituting decaffeinated coffee and grain-based coffee substitutes. You can gradually phase out the decaffeinated coffee until a point is reached where only caffeine-free coffee substitute is being drunk. The same method can be used to reduce cups of tea by slowly introducing herb or fruit teas that are appealing.

If alcohol intake is too high or too frequent, it can be helpful to give yourself a couple of alcohol-free weeks, choosing palatable alternatives such as sparkling mineral water with a twist of lemon or lime, or a sparkling herbal drink with added natural fruit flavouring. When going out for a drink with friends try a non-alcoholic cocktail. These look and taste the same as the alcoholic variety, but without the drawbacks. After the two alcohol-free weeks, establish a pattern of always staying well under your weekly alcohol unit allowance.

Making sure enough essential fatty acids are included in the diet

Many of us may think that we should be on radically low fat diets in order to look after our bodies the best we can. While it is true that we generally eat far too much fat in our diets in the Western world (due to the emphasis on fast foods, snacks and refined foods), there are important fats that can play a vital role in encouraging optimum hormone balance in our bodies. These 'good guys' cannot be manufactured by our bodies and, as a result, we must include enough of them in our daily intake of food if we are to enjoy the maximum possibility of good health.

These important fats are called essential fatty acids (EFAs) and they provide the basic building blocks that are needed for our bodies to carry out a host of functions. If a deficiency of EFAs occurs, the result can be a detrimental effect on our hormonal balance, which can lead to extra problems at menopause. Too low an intake of EFAs can lead to problems with aggravation of PMS-type symptoms, fluid retention, poor skin and hair quality, poor liver function, slow-healing wounds, heart problems, vaginal dryness and arthritic joints.

If we change to a drastically low-fat, unbalanced diet our bodies respond by shutting down ovarian function. This is done in response to our bodies getting the message that too little nutritious food is being ingested, so a full-term pregnancy cannot be supported. Once we have ceased to ovulate, we are far more likely to experience oestrogen dominance (see Chapter 6, 'The Pros and Cons of Hormone Replacement Therapy', for an explanation of why this is of particular relevance to us as we approach and move beyond menopause). On the other hand, increasing any old type of fat won't solve the problem, since we need to know which fats are health-promoting, and which fats are a health hazard.

The nature of the fat that we eat has a direct effect on prostaglandin production in the body which plays a vital role in regulating blood pressure and inflammatory processes in our bodies. If we have a healthy supply of 'good' fats from oily fish and olive oil this will encourage balanced prostaglandin production. Unhealthy fats, however, such as hydrogenated fats in margarines will result in an excess of prostaglandin production which can aggravate fluid retention, inflammation, and general PMS-type problems such as severe mood swings. 'Bad' fats to watch out for include any oils that have a reputation for being readily oxidised such as corn, safflower, peanut and sunflower oils. The problem with these oils is that they are chemically unstable, which leaves them easily transformed into carriers of free radicals when heated to high temperatures and exposed to oxygen. Free radicals are rampaging molecules that act rather like terrorists within our bodies when they occur in excess, leading to damage of cell membranes, proteins, and even DNA. Hydrogenated fats (vegetable oils that are treated in order to make them solid at room temperature) are known to contribute to free radical production and should be best avoided.

One of the unwelcome consequences of a hefty or regular intake of foods made from hydrogenated fats is an increased risk of heart and circulatory disorders due to the way that free radicals appear to damage the delicate lining of blood vessels. This then encourages the build-up of fatty plaques that can eventually clog up our arteries, leading to chronic hypertension, and may leave us vulnerable to an elevated risk of heart attacks and strokes. Saturated fats which are naturally solid at room temperature such as cheese, butter, and red meat bring similar problems since they encourage the storing of fat deposits which our bodies cannot break down. As a basic rule of thumb, the harder saturated fat is at room temperature, the greater the likelihood that it will form undesirable deposits in our arteries leaving them in a hardened and clogged state. In addition, saturated fats can also contribute to the malabsorption of EFAs.

Too frequent use of unstable polyunsaturated fats such as refined sunflower oils that are made using exposure to extremely high temperatures (as opposed to a cold-pressed method) may also raise our risk of developing breast cancer. The good news, however, is that if we choose our oils wisely (such as using monounsaturated, cold-pressed, virgin olive oil) we can positively protect our hearts and circulatory systems. Additional sources of healthy unsaturated fats include seeds, nuts, oily fish, and vegetables.

EFAs fall into two basic categories of monounsaturated oils (such as olive oil) and polyunsaturated oils (such as sunflower oil). Within these two categories there is an additional split into omega 3 fatty acids that are found in fish oils, linseeds, pumpkin seeds, walnuts and green, leafy vegetables; and omega 6 oils that can be found in corn, sesame, unrefined safflower, and sunflower oils. Omega 3 oils often lacking in our diets are of particular importance for us at menopause as they can help guard against heart attacks and strokes. They can also enhance immune system function, speed up our metabolic rate, and boost energy levels as well as balancing prostaglandin production.

If you are concerned about increasing your intake of EFAs the following basic advice will be helpful:

- Always use virgin, cold-pressed olive oil for salad dressing and in cooking.

- Avoid hydrogenated fats wherever possible, making sure that you *never* use hydrogenated margarine for frying – always opt for cold-pressed olive oil or a little butter instead.
- Alternative oils that can be used in salad dressings include unrefined sunflower, safflower, or sesame oils. Take care to buy or store them in dark glass containers, and always store them in the fridge since they go rancid very readily.
- Have regular, plentiful portions of oily fish such as mackerel, sardines, or salmon.
- Make a point of enjoying fresh, unroasted, unsalted nuts such as walnuts, brazils and almonds as a regular snack. Avoid nuts that have been fried or roasted, since they will probably have been fried in refined oils and are also likely to have a hefty portion of salt added to them.
- Try tahini (made from creamed sesame seeds) on salads, or in sauces and dressings.

Including soya products

A great deal of interest is currently being generated around the use of plant-based oestrogen (phytoestrogen) for the relief of common menopausal symptoms such hot flushes. Studies are currently under way in order to examine how helpful phyt-oestrogens may also be in protecting and improving bone density, as well as protecting against heart and circulatory disease. It is now recognised that women who eat a diet that is rich in phyt-oestrogens (such as the Japanese) appear to experience far fewer problems and trauma with menopause, while in addition they incur a reduced risk of breast cancer or heart disease.

Phytoestrogens fall into two main types: lignans which can be obtained from linseeds and wheat bran, and isoflavones which can be obtained from soya. Isoflavones are currently the focus of special interest because of the way that they appear to mimic the protective effects of oestrogen (in guarding against loss of bone density), while at the same time protecting against the negative effect that oestro-gen can have in stimulating breast cells. As a result, judicious use of phytoestrogens may have a significant role to play in protecting us against hormone-related conditions such as breast cancer, heart disease, osteoporosis and menopausal problems.

In contrast to the average Japanese daily intake of isoflavones (approximately 80 g) we in the West are lucky if we get around 1 g from our daily food intake. It has been estimated that we need to aim for around 45 g if we want to obtain maximum relief from menopausal symptoms. This should be easily done by including a couple of glasses of soya milk a day (making sure that it's GM-free), or a healthy portion of tofu. Additional sources could include textured vegetable protein (soya-based), miso (seasoning for soups or stocks made from fermented bean paste), soya, kidney or aduki beans, lentils, chickpeas, and products made from soya flour.

Including anti-oxidant nutrients in your diet

Anti-oxidant nutrients are essential allies in protecting us against the negative effects of free radicals which can leave us open to increased risk of heart disease, signs of early ageing, and degenerative diseases such as arthritis. Anti-oxidant nutrients are to be found in foods that are rich in beta-carotene (a precursor to vitamin A), vitamin C, and vitamin E. We should be especially vigilant about increasing our intake of anti-oxidants if any of the following apply to us:

* Regular exposure to radiation from the sun.
* We smoke, or drink alcohol.
* Exposure to high levels of atmospheric pollution.
* Regular intake of processed, convenience, or fried foods.
* High levels of psychological and physical stress.

Beta-carotene has a double function: on the one hand, the body can convert it to vitamin A, and what is left over acts as an anti-oxidant. Foods that are rich in beta-carotene are easy to spot since they tend to be any fruit or vegetable that is bright yellow or orange in colour, such as carrots, mangoes, apricots, peaches or sweet potatoes. Deep green coloured vegetables such as spinach, parsley, watercress, asparagus, or broccoli can also provide us with rich sources of this basic nutrient.

Vitamin C is a powerful anti-oxidant nutrient that is a vital ally in combating the damaging effect of free radicals in the body. It is to be found in the fluid that flows between our cells, acting as a 'search-and-destroy' agent dealing with any free radicals that are unfortunate enough to cross its path. However, it can be difficult to obtain enough of this vitamin on a daily basis, because it is extremely easily destroyed on exposure to the air (a process called oxidation), or during cooking processes such as boiling. As a result, take care when cooking vegetables to chop them just before cooking so that their vitamin C content has a reduced chance of oxidising and evaporating into the atmosphere.

Vitamin C-rich foods include any of the following: black-currants, parsley, raw green peppers, strawberries, watercress, sprouts, lemons, oranges, broccoli, grapefruit and cauliflower.

Vitamin E has been described as the most important anti-oxidant nutrient because it can protect the fats that surround every cell in the body. It is also of vital importance in supporting the efficient working of our immune systems because of the way it can strengthen white blood cells in their fight against infection. It has also been suggested that vitamin E may play an important role in discouraging the development of heart disease and circulatory problems. Vitamin E works in tandem with vitamin C in neutralising free radicals in our bodies, so we should ideally be making sure that we have optimum quantities of both in our diet.

The main sources for vitamin E are vegetable oils (wheat germ, sunflower or safflower), nuts and whole grains. Always bear in mind that this vitamin is readily lost through any refining or processing (for instance the refining process that is necessary to make white flour). Vitamin E can also be destroyed when it comes in contact with oxygen in the air, warmth or sunlight. As a result, always store vegetable oils in a fridge or a cool, dark cupboard, making sure that the tops of bottles are kept firmly secured when not in use.

Cooking methods can also adversely affect vitamin E content, with shallow or deep frying causing the major problems. Apart from other drawbacks of deep frying (such as saturating food in excess fat and stimulating the production of free radicals), it can also destroy up to 90 per cent of vitamin E content. This is an even greater possibility if the cooking oil has become rancid by storing it in warm conditions.

So, to summarise the basic advice given so far, if we want to eat for maximum health at menopause we should be aiming to follow these general guidelines:

- Eat from as wide a range of fresh, healthy food as possible in order to make sure that food does not become repetitive, monotonous or boring. By eating as varied a diet as possible, there is a greater chance that a broader complement of nutrients is going to be available to us, so that we are less likely to find that nutritional imbalances occur.
- Always avoid drastic eating regimes that involve undereating or overeating since this is likely to contribute to problems with hormone imbalances. If we have a low body weight, or move from bingeing to starvation in a desperate effort to keep slim, we are substantially increasing our risks of more severe menopausal symptoms (as a result of lowered oestrogen secretion) as well as running greater risks of suffering from osteoporosis. The risk factor rises proportionally yet again if we are smokers or drink more than moderate amounts of alcohol.
- A significant proportion of our diets should be made up of high-fibre foods including whole grains, fresh, raw fruit and vegetables.
- Avoid foods that are high in hydrogenated or saturated fats.
- Ideal foods should be low in sodium and refined sugar.
- Alcohol should be drunk in strictly regulated amounts.
- Concentrate on eating whole grains, oily fish, organic poultry, beans, pulses, organic fruit, raw, organic vegetables, soya products, and a small amount of organic dairy food.

Eating for healthy bones

There is little wonder that osteoporosis is a problem that is causing growing anxiety and concern in many women who are approaching or beyond menopausal age, since it has a reputation as a 'silent' condition that we are unlikely to be aware of until a fracture actually occurs. However, questions have been raised about the inevitability of osteoporosis occurring as part and parcel of the menopausal process, since maximum bone density is reached for most women while we are in our mid-thirties when oestrogen levels are still high. It may be more appropriate to regard osteoporosis as a condition that can be symptomatic of a culmination of years of a poor diet, sedentary, stressful lifestyle, and a preoccupation with drastic weight loss plans.

In order to have healthy, strong, resilient bones it appears that a healthy diet, appropriate exercise, and sensible use of nutritional supplements are the most powerful allies we have at our disposal. Strong bones need a balanced supply of the basic building blocks which include calcium, vitamin D, vitamin A and phosphorus. It helps to remember that calcium is not just needed in order to keep our bones resilient and strong, since it plays an important role in allowing our muscles to contract as well as helping to regulate blood pressure.

Of course, nutrients should be initially obtained wherever possible from a healthy diet, in order to avoid pill-popping as a way of pasting over the cracks of a negligent or positively unhealthy diet. It also helps to bear in mind that while diet may be the most important topic to discuss when we are looking at the problem of osteoporosis, it is only one important perspective on protecting the health of our bones. Other aspects of our lifestyles that also have a major impact on bone density that must not be overlooked include eliminating smoking, while also drastically cutting down on alcohol consumption. As a result, we should be aiming to adopt a multi-faceted support system in order to keep our bone density at an optimum level for as long as possible rather than just popping a calcium supplement and hoping that may be enough to do the trick.

When calcium supplements are used within a broadly based approach to protecting bone density they can make a substantial difference, since a study that was published in the *New England Journal of Medicine* in 1993 revealed that appropriate use of calcium supplements can reduce decalcification of bone by roughly half. It is also true that some of us may struggle to get enough calcium from our daily diets and may benefit from a booster dose in the form of a supplement. However, not all calcium supplements are equal, and it is helpful to be aware that other nutrients (such as magnesium and vitamin D) are also required in order to maximise the chance of calcium utilisation and absorption.

Although calcium carbonate is the most commonly available calcium supplement, it is poorly absorbed by the body and can lead to digestive problems, increased possibility of kidney stone formation, arthritic joints, and nodules in breast tissue. Calcium citrate, on the other hand, although containing a lower dose in each tablet, does tend to be more readily absorbed by the body and is generally less likely to lead to unwanted side effects. Also bear in mind that magnesium, vitamin C and vitamin D also play a vital role in assisting our bodies to metabolise calcium. We should be aiming for a basic ratio of twice as much magnesium as calcium for maximum possibility of absorption to take place. Good dietary sources of magnesium are apples, seeds, nuts, figs, lemons and green vegetables.

Vitamin D can be obtained from exposure to sunlight as well as from dietary sources. This nutrient plays a vitally important role in supporting the absorption of calcium and phosphorus in bony tissue. As a result, a deficiency of vitamin D can contribute to calcium leaching from our bones, leaving them more vulnerable to becoming porous and brittle. Rich dietary sources include oily fish and fish oils.

Always guard against the temptation to think that if a little of something is beneficial then more must be even better, especially with regard to taking supplements. Taking a higher dose of calcium than the body needs can result in any of the following: constipation, abdominal bloating, and poor absorption of other minerals including iron and zinc.

Dietary sources of calcium

Most of us will be aware by now that calcium can be readily obtained from dairy products. It is important, however, to bear in mind that there are additional non-dairy calcium sources in the form of spinach, tofu, dark green vegetables, seeds, nuts, fish eaten with the bones intact (such as sardines) and beans. It also helps to remember that we are unlikely to benefit from increasing the amount of available calcium in our diets if we are still taking regular amounts of food or drinks that contribute to increasing excretion of calcium from our bones. Items to cut out, or drastic-ally cut down in order to maximise calcium conservation include coffee, strong tea, chocolate, fizzy drinks, alcohol, cigarettes, and excessive amounts of animal protein.

It is important to take into consideration that even within the food items mentioned above certain items are more beneficial when eaten in large amounts than others. For instance, if we eat a high proportion of protein foods that have an acidic effect when digested (such as milk, cheese, red meat, chicken and fish) calcium reserves are drawn from our bones and teeth in order to balance the situation. Coffee also has an acidic effect on the system, and it has been estimated that drinking anything over three cups a day can increase our risk of developing osteoporosis by as much as 82 per cent. On the other hand, items that have the opposite alkaline effect (fruit and vegetables) do not promote de-calcification of bone.

Eating for a healthy heart

Many of us are likely to be aware of the vital role that lifestyle factors play in protecting us against, or leaving us vulnerable to, heart disease. Few of us can have missed the strong negative messages that have been given out with regard to the dangers of smoking, poor stress-management, high blood pressure, a sedent-ary lifestyle, being overweight, and a diet that is high in saturated fats. We may also know that women are substantially less likely to suffer from heart disease before they experience menopause, but that this risk rises substantially once menopause has occurred.

It has been suggested that HRT gives us valuable protection against heart disease in our post-menopausal years, but studies so far appear to show contradictory results. See the 'Heart health and HRT' section in Chapter 6 (p. 121) for a more general explanation of why it may not be wise to depend too much on HRT to help us prevent heart disease. Reducing our risk of developing heart and circulatory problems may be viewed from a very similar perspective to preventing osteoporosis. In other words, we have the best chance of avoiding both serious conditions if we adopt a number of positive factors into our lifestyles, rather than relying solely on medication to sort potential problems out.

Although cigarettes are not a food, we should always start with a discussion of the importance of giving up smoking when we are considering how to do our best to protect the condition of our hearts and our circulatory systems. Smokers run more than twice the risk of having a heart attack than non-smokers, while cigarette smoking is the highest risk factor in predisposing us towards sudden death from a cardiac episode. If we are smokers with a tendency to high blood pressure and are significantly overweight, our risk factor rises substantially.

To make matters worse, we have already mentioned how smoking increases our risk of developing osteoporosis due to the negative effect smoking has on oestrogen secretion. As a result, when we smoke we are significantly elevating our risk of developing the two most serious conditions associated with menopause: osteoporosis and heart disease. On the other hand, if we make a concerted effort to kick the habit, we can at a single stroke considerably reduce our risk of developing two major menopausal problems, while at the same time leaving ourselves less vulnerable to additional diseases such as lung cancer or bronchitis.

The cholesterol question

A great deal of attention has been focused on the connection between intake of foods that are high in cholesterol and a predisposition to heart disease. However, it now appears that intake of dietary cholesterol does not necessarily translate neatly into levels of cholesterol that are to be found circulating in the bloodstream. Our blood cholesterol levels may have more to do with the way in which our bodies process the foods we ingest, rather than only being related to the amount of cholesterol-rich foods included in our diets.

The way in which we process cholesterol is affected by the way high density lipoprotein (HDL) and low density lipoprotein (LDL) work in our bodies. If we have too high a level of LDL and too low a level of HDL, we are at significant risk of developing hardening and narrowing of our artery walls, which in turn leaves us at proportionally greater risk of developing heart disease. It has also been suggested that rather than focusing solely on cholesterol as the 'bad guy' in relation to raising our risk of developing heart disease, we should be even more concerned about cutting down the amount of saturated fats that we eat. This is due to the emerging evidence that suggests saturated fats may play a greater role than cholesterol in predisposing us to the development of heart problems.

Hydrogenated fats can also play an extremely negative role in encouraging degenerative conditions such as hardening of the arteries and heart disease, and for this reason are best avoided. On the other hand, essential fatty acids that are to be found in oily fish, nuts, seeds and monounsaturated oils such as olive oil play an important positive role in protecting us against heart disease. If we feel we want to reduce our blood cholesterol levels, the fatty acids found in these foods will help us do this, while also discouraging an excessive tendency to coagulation of the blood and reducing our risk of furred-up arteries. We should also bear in mind that problems associated with hydrogenated fats are linked to the production of free radicals in the body, a process that can be reduced by making sure that we have an adequate supply of anti-oxidant nutrients in order to combat the degenerative processes that free radicals can promote.

If we are concerned about the health of our hearts and circulatory systems, the following measures should be adopted as part of an overall heart protection plan:

• Increase the amount of fresh vegetables, fruits, unroasted nuts and seeds eaten on a daily basis.

- Introduce soya products that are rich in phytoestrogens to the diet, since these can help protect us against hot flushes, osteoporosis and heart disease. Using soya beans in cooking can also be an invaluable way of obtaining an important form of protein without the saturated fat hazard of proteins obtained from dairy foods.
- Avoid saturated and hydrogenated fats such as cheese, full-fat milk, red meat, and margarines that use the process of hydrogenation to make refined vegetable oil solid at room temperature.
- Give up smoking for all of the reasons listed above.
- Exercise regularly in order to give the heart and lungs a healthy workout and keep the circulatory system moving.
- Consider supplementing with nutrients that have a reputation for supporting the health of the heart and circulatory system. These include vitamin E, vitamin C, linseed oil capsules, and magnesium.
- If you are carrying a great deal of excess weight around the waist and belly, make a concerted effort to tone up and reduce the amount of flesh carried on these areas by exercising. This is significant because the way in which our fat reserves are distributed appears to have an impact on how much we are at risk of developing heart problems. If we have a classic British 'pear shape' with any excess inches being carried on the lower half of the body, we may be frustrated at not having slender thighs, but the good news is that we are at a statistically lower risk of suffering from heart disease. On the other hand, if we an 'apple shape' and carry a significant amount of extra flesh on our waists and belly, we are at greater risk of developing cardiac problems. As with high blood pressure, a sedentary existence, or a diet that is high in saturated fat, having a male-type pattern of fat distribution may not on its own lead to a heart attack. However, if it is combined with a range of additional high-risk factors with regard to heart health, it may be the last straw that tips the balance against us.
- Most of all, always bear in mind that we stand the best chance of keeping a healthy heart and circulatory system if we take an

active, positive stance. By adopting the general strategies given above, in combination with the lifestyle changes mentioned in Chapter 3, 'Preparation for Menopause', we can feel empowered to make the most of our health as we approach this vital watershed. This has to be a more positive situation than regarding problems with our hearts and circulatory systems as an inevitable part of moving on to a new phase in our lives.

To supplement or not to supplement?

Vitamin and mineral supplements are hot news these days, with one formula after another appearing on the market. These tablets and capsules are seen by many to hold out promises with regard to correcting important imbalances in our systems, and boosting everything from our energy levels to our libido. Opinions vary hugely on the need for supplements, with the diehard sceptics suggesting that this is no more than a racket that trades on our insecurity, and convinces us to buy unnecessary nutrients that we should all be getting from a basic diet. At the other extreme, we have opinions that claim we live in such a polluted, stressful and nutritionally compromised world that we must judiciously boost our flagging nutritional status with a wide range of supplements.

The sensible answer would seem to lie somewhere between these two extreme views, since we always have to take individual circumstances into the equation before we can judge how appropriate a course of action is likely to be. There are undoubtedly specific situations where well-selected nutritional supplements can make a definite difference to overall health and vitality. These include any of the following:

- Environments where we know we are exposed to low-grade pollution, chemical emissions, and environmental toxins on a regular basis: this would include most offices where we may be in the same room as photocopiers or faxes, and where computer monitors are on all day. The situation may be compromised even more if air conditioning or central heating units are used

inefficiently, or not maintained as often as necessary.
- Particularly stressful phases of life where we may have been presented with physical and emotional challenges over an extended period of time.
- Times of life where we may have been neglecting the quality of our daily diet due to extreme short-term pressure of work, or changes in family routine.
- Developmental milestones where our bodies may be drawing more than usual on our reserves of energy and vitality. This would include the phases of puberty, pregnancy and menopause.
- Taking conventional medication that can affect the delicate nutritional balance of our bodies. For instance, drugs such as diuretics can result in the body losing potassium, while antibiotics kill off friendly bacteria in the gut as well as the ones they are attempting to eradicate. The end result can be digestive disturbance that can lead to malabsorption of nutrients.

As we can see from the above categories, menopause is one of the specific situations where it may be wise to consider using an appropriately selected programme of supplements in order to give us a nutritional boost. This may be especially the case if approaching menopause is combined with a number of the other categories on the list, including an unhealthy work environment, or exposure to additional stress. On the other hand, if we have an excellent record of health, eat a varied, balanced diet made up of fresh foods that embraces most of the advice given above, and if we are at very low risk of developing problems with osteoporosis, we may find that our nutritional needs are being generally met already and we may not need to look any further unless we become unduly stressed.

However, if we are aware that as we have been approaching menopause we have become fatigued, inclined to develop recurrent infections, with a less than ideal diet through professional or domestic circumstances, we should seriously consider improving our nutritional status by initially using appropriate supplements while we get to grips with getting our daily eating plan sorted out.

The following section provides a quick summary of some of the nutrients that we are most in need of as we approach, and move beyond, menopause. These are the basic building blocks that we must have in adequate supply if we are to feel fit, energised, focused and resilient as we move beyond this exciting watershed. In addition, the combination of nutrients needed to protect our bones, muscles and heart are also mentioned so that we can make sure that we are making the best choices with regard to protecting and nurturing our physical health.

As always, try to make sure that the basic nutritional support comes from a high-quality, healthy diet, adding in extra help from supplements when needed. This tends to be a more positive approach than paying too little attention to our daily diets and relying too much on nutritional supplements as a damage limitation exercise. After all, if we are attempting to take a genuinely holistic approach to building better health from within, we will always need to take the long-term approach which ultimately gives us the power to radically change our lives physically, emotionally and mentally. One we have the chance to experience the benefits of this course of action we are unlikely to want to settle for less.

Anti-ageing nutrients at a glance

Calcium

This is the first nutrient we all tend to think of in relation to preserving bone density and strong, healthy teeth. However, it also plays an essential role in balancing blood-clotting mechanisms, helps prevent muscle cramps, lowers blood cholesterol levels, balances blood pressure, and may also have an important part to play in helping us achieve a healthy, sound sleep.

Dietary sources include soya beans, dairy products, tinned fish eaten with the bones intact, pulses, sesame seeds, and green, leafy vegetables.

Recommended dosages can range from 800 to 2,000 mg daily.

Greater chance of absorption occurs if calcium is taken in combination with magnesium (in a two-to-one ratio). It also helps to take calcium supplements in smaller doses twice or three times through the day with meals.

Beta-carotene

This precursor of vitamin A is one of the major anti-oxidant nutrients. Because of its ability to counteract the damaging effect of free radical activity, it is one of the most powerful allies we have in preventing the signs of early ageing and protecting us against the development of degenerative disease.

Dietary sources include dark green vegetables, and bright yellow, red, and orange fruit and vegetables.

The recommended daily allowance is 15 mg per day.

Vitamin D

This is absolutely vital for the body to enjoy maximum use and absorption of calcium and other minerals. As a result, vitamin D plays a vital role in protecting and maintaining the health and strength of teeth, bones and gums.

Dietary sources include fish and fish oils. Some vitamin D is also acquired through exposure to sunlight.

The recommended daily allowance is 350 iu daily.

Vitamin C

Vitamin C is another vital anti-oxidant nutrient that protects the health of our teeth and gums, and maintains elasticity and youthful texture of the skin. It also plays an essential role in assisting the body in combating infection by boosting immune-system functioning and encouraging absorption of iron.

Dietary sources include citrus fruit, berries (strawberries, blackberries, etc.), potatoes and green leafy vegetables.

The recommended daily allowance is 70 mg per day, but nutritionists may often recommend doses of 1–2 g per day.

Vitamin B complex

This group of nutrients plays an essential role in supporting the health of the nervous system, something that becomes of special importance when we are under protracted physical, emotional or mental stress.

Dietary sources include pulses, nuts, whole grains and products made from whole grains (such as bread or pasta), soya beans and fortified cereals.

The suggested daily allowance is 50 mg of B1, B2, B3, and B6 with 200 mcg of folic acid. It is best to take to take B vitamins together in the form of a B Complex supplement, since they appear to work most effectively when taken in this way.

Vitamin E

This is the third important anti-oxidant nutrient which plays a vital role in protecting the health of the heart and circulatory system, as well as preventing signs of damage and early ageing to the skin as a result of free radical activity.

Dietary sources include vegetable oils, seeds, nuts, wheatgerm and dark green vegetables.

The recommended daily allowance is 15–30 iu (international unit) but most nutritionists may suggest 100–200 iu per day.

Boron

This is a trace element that is considered to play a role of vital importance in boosting flagging oestrogen levels as well as reducing decalcification of bone. Boron appears to improve the metabolism of the minerals calcium, phosphorus and magnesium, while also supporting the manufacture of vitamin D which also enhances absorption of calcium.

Dietary sources include alfalfa, cabbage, dark green leafy vegetables and kelp.

The suggested dose where bone density is a problem: 2–8 mg a day.

Selenium

This is a vital anti-oxidant nutrient and immune system booster which prevents signs of early ageing and recurrent infections. It also works in tandem with vitamin E to protect the health of the heart.

Dietary sources include sea vegetables, red meat, shellfish, wheat germ, brown rice and nuts.

The recommended daily allowance is 50–200 mcg per day.

Magnesium

This mineral plays a vital role in promoting optimum functioning of the heart, as well as promoting maximum utilisation and absorption of calcium, and converting sugars into energy. Magnesium can be a vital ally in acting as a natural tranquilliser as well as discouraging the build-up of fatty plaques in arteries. A deficiency of magnesium can give rise to decalcification of the bones as well as premature loss of skin tone, mood swings, muscle cramps, and poor metabolism.

Dietary sources include seafood, apples, seaweeds, tofu and sesame seeds.

The recommended daily allowance is 350 mg per day. Since magnesium is known to have an effect on the kidneys and heart, seek medical advice before embarking on taking a supplement, if you suffer from heart or kidney disorders.

5

Moving On Up: the Basic Benefits of Exercise

When we speak of 'freeing the body' it helps enormously to remember we have the most powerful tool at our disposal in regular exercise. Apart from building increased confidence in our physical capabilities, regular, enjoyable exercise also provides us with a sense of exhilaration and freedom that cannot easily be found elsewhere.

In addition, physical activity brings an extremely positive bonus with it in the form of 'freeing the mind', since positive emotional benefits are now known to be experienced by those of us who maintain a healthy approach to physical fitness. Plenty of attention has also been drawn to the stress-busting benefits that have been attributed to regular, vigorous exercise, or combining physical movement with relaxation techniques as we can do in yoga. As we can see, exercise is one of the pivotal allies we should make maximum use of if we are to enjoy optimum physical, emotional and mental well-being and vitality.

At no time is this more relevant than when we are approaching menopause, since this experience allows us maximum opportunity for re-evaluation, provided, of course, we are willing to take it. If we have previously considered ourselves physically unfit, considering the advent of menopause can be the very incentive we need to get into optimum physical shape.

Most writers would agree that there is nothing quite like an imminent deadline to get them moving. Contemplating menopause can fulfil a similar function, bringing home the important message that we do not have endless time within which to make positive changes. So, instead of putting off taking up exercise, we need to take on board the fact that the sooner we do it the faster we will see the positive benefits, that can have such a significant impact on the sort of menopause we experience.

There is also the additional freedom exercise will bring us from the aches and pains that are not inevitable at mid-life. After all, these problems are often mistakenly associated with getting older, rather than being seen as an indication of the cumulative effect of an unhealthy lifestyle.

Body maintenance

If we take the mechanical analogy that we have already used in the nutrition chapter and develop it further, we can see that we can apply the same basic principles to our bodies as to our cars. Just as we can't afford to mishandle a car by driving it into the ground, so also, and even more emphatically, in the case of our bodies, a lifetime of unhealthy wear and tear is inevitably going to show up in joint problems and other limitations in movement. On the other hand, in the same way that a car which is left completely idle and neglected will quickly develop a flat battery and begin to seize up, the same is true of our bodies. A completely sedentary lifestyle will make us feel fatigued and generally stiff and unfit.

What we are ideally looking for is an appropriate amount of exercise and physical effort that gives us the optimum amount of challenge required to keep our bodies energised and in generally great shape. Too extreme and strenuous an approach can be as bad as too little activity, since the key word is the same in this chapter as in every other section of the book: balance.

When we employ a balanced approach to exercise we will be giving our bodies enough physical activity to improve bone density, and our hearts and circulatory systems a healthy workout, while also increasing flexibility and strength in our muscles and joints. After a balanced exercise programme, we should feel our energy levels are increased rather than depleted. In addition, we should also find that we are generally less stressed and tense, while also enjoying the benefits of being more emotionally calm and resilient.

It is being increasingly acknowledged that the benefits of regular, enjoyable exercise have a particular relevance for us as we reach mid-life. Important as it is to be physically active when we are in our twenties, we can get away with an awful lot at this time and not seem to pay a price. This is as true with regard to what we eat and drink, as with the amount of exercise we take, since a youthful body can appear to be infinitely forgiving and resilient. This is not true in reality, since we can do plenty of damage through an unhealthy lifestyle when we are younger – it's just that the results take longer to show up. However, once we have reached our thirties and move into our forties, it's a different story.

It has been suggested that the ravages of a severely unhealthy way of living are most likely to become obvious by the time we hit the middle phase of our fifth decade. The very welcome good news, however, is that those of us who have made an effort to get ourselves as fit and healthy as we can from our thirties onwards, will begin to reap obvious benefits by the time we are cruising into our forties and fifties. These advantages become clear in a range of positive qualities including enviable energy levels, improved strength, greater physical stamina, and ease of movement.

Making exercise one of the mainstays of our daily routine appears to be one of the major ways we can prepare ourselves for a fit and active life beyond menopause. A recent study conducted in Boston revealed that women who took part in a strength-training programme for a period of twelve months actually reversed their course of ageing by anything up to twenty years. In other words, their bone mass and muscle strength and bulk were increased, while their heart rates were lowered, and their body shapes became more sculpted.

It is also extremely heartening to appreciate that, with the less competitive and more holistic trends in exercise techniques that have become popular in the latter half of the 1990s (yoga, t'ai chi, and Pilates), there are few obstacles that prevent us becoming fit at whatever age we choose to start. Sadly, this was something we could not say about the approaches to exercise that became fashionable in the 1980s, since phrases like 'going for the burn' and 'no pain, no gain' led far too many of us down the road of injury and ill health because of a desperate desire to show that we could compete with others.

Thankfully, the current emphasis is quite different, with much more of a tendency to encourage us to work to the maximum of our capacity for strength and stamina, but never to push ourselves to the point where we are aware that we are causing ourselves pain. After all, severe pain is the basic mechanism that our bodies have to alert us to the fact that all is not well. If we ignore extreme pain when we exercise, we do this at our peril.

On the other hand, if we work within our basic fitness boundaries, building stamina, and challenging ourselves without causing pain or injury, we are likely to gain an increased sense of physical awareness that can protect us from tackling any physical demand that may not be appropriate for us. This basic skill is often referred to as an ability to tune in and listen to our bodies, something that should never be lost sight of whenever we are taxing ourselves physically.

Freedom from boundaries

One of the most refreshing aspects of the way we consider exercise these days is the sheer range of activities open to us once we decide we want to get fit. So, if we have been carrying around the feeling that we must inevitably be an unfit adult, with no choice except to be a couch potato because we were a shockingly unfit child, this is no longer a viable excuse.

I know this to be true, since I was exactly the sort of child who was overweight, lacking in co-ordination, and hugely unsuited to the only two games on offer at school: hockey and netball. Every Wednesday afternoon I was to be found hiding in the spartan changing rooms, hoping to goodness that no one would notice that I was missing. Of course, they did, and I would emerge on to a freezing, exposed hockey pitch, wondering how on earth I could possibly endure the next two hours of punishment.

The sheer physical discomfort and sense of painful humiliation did nothing to make me gain a sense of confidence in my body. This was something that I was to discover much later when the fitness craze of the eighties made it impossible to ignore the aerobics studios. Although it has emerged that there were plenty of negative aspects to eighties-style fitness classes (as we have seen above), they did plenty of people like myself a huge favour in encouraging them to explore exercise as an option, possibly for the first time in their lives.

There will be countless stories similar to mine, where someone who was written off as physically unfit as a child has discovered, to their joy, that they are not condemned to this sense of physical weakness and inferiority for life. There are plenty of examples of women who have taken up yoga in their sixties, who have gained a sense of physical, mental and emotional equilibrium that they would not have thought possible.

Role models such as Leslie Kenton write extremely persuasively of the sheer exhilaration of discovering the joy of running or weight training at a later stage. When in doubt, always remember it's never to late to act on your impulses and get fit; it's taking the first step that is usually the most difficult part.

Fringe benefits of body conditioning at menopause

We can reap positive benefit from getting fit at any age, and in many ways it's very healthy to adopt the attitude that developing physical fitness is never wasted. However, there are specific advantages that we can experience if we take up regular exercise as we approach menopause.

In an ideal situation we should begin a physical fitness programme in our early thirties, since this is roughly the age at which we have reached maximum bone density. In addition, our hormone levels can become prone to fluctuation any time from our mid-thirties onwards, so this is an optimum stage to make a regular exercise programme part of our lives.

As we can see from the following information, it really is worth making the effort to get moving, since the potential benefits that we can gain cover an impressively broad spectrum. This is surprisingly wide in scope, and ranges from the relief of specific symptoms associated with menopause, to promotion of increased emotional and physical resilience and balance.

- Greater life expectancy: even if we only do one hour of exercise a week we can reduce our risk of death by as much as 24 per cent.
- Improved energy levels: it has been suggested that women of menopausal age who exercise on a regular basis have 25 per cent more energy than couch potatoes.
- Faster metabolic rate: when we exercise regularly we can boost our basal metabolic rate (the rate at which we burn up our food to provide energy and warmth) by as much as 8 per cent. As a result, we are far more likely to be able to maintain a healthy body weight.
- Increased heart health: because our hearts are made of muscle they are designed to be used and worked out. As a result, it appears that we can decrease our risk of developing heart disease if we become physically active through engaging in a regular exercise programme.
- Controlled food cravings: many of us may have experienced the way in which exercise can take the edge off too large an appetite. These effects do not diminish as we approach and move beyond menopause, since it has been reported that women of menopausal age who are physically fit, experience significantly reduced cravings for two of the greatest health hazards and the focus of addictive eating patterns: sweet and fatty foods.

- Improved bone density and strength: evidence suggests that those of us who continue to be physically active have significantly healthier bone density than those of us who have a sedentary lifestyle. This may be partly connected to the way in which exercise has a positive effect on oestrogen secretion.
- Greater emotional balance: since regular, rhythmic exercise encourages the secretion of endorphins which make us feel calmer and more positive, those of us who enjoy physical exercise are likely to be less prone to depression and mood swings at menopause.
- Fewer hot flushes: partly because of its positive effect on oestrogen secretion, regular exercise brings measurable benefits to those of us who want to avoid the problems of hot flushes and night sweats. It has been suggested getting physically fit can reduce a tendency to hot flushes by approximately 50 per cent.

Exercise and bone density

As we have already established, the question of how to protect against brittle bones (osteoporosis) after menopause is one of the major issues that clued-up women have to face. However, the good news is that exercise can make a significant positive difference to bone density. This effect is further enhanced when it is adopted as a regular feature of our lives, combined with a range of additional supportive measures. These include an effective stress-reduction plan, and nutritious diet that provides us with the basic balanced approach that we need to maintain maximum bone density.

Forms of exercise that have a particularly beneficial effect on bone density include brisk walking, tennis, aerobics, badminton and yoga. For maximum benefit, the ideal form of physical activity needs to exert pressure on the bones without exerting excessive pressure on the joints. This is why jogging on a hard surface may be problematic. Although it is a weight-bearing activity, it does involve the potential drawback of harsh, pounding movements that can have a damaging effect on the easily injured knee and ankle joints.

If jogging is a particular favourite, it may be worth considering jogging on the spot on a rebounder, since the surface provides a cushioning effect that can help guard against joint injuries. When it is done on a regular basis, rebounding also appears to have a beneficial effect in stimulating the immune system.

The benefits of appropriate exercise in protecting bone density have been revealed in an interesting study. It was discovered that women who took a brisk walk four times a week, lasting fifty minutes, increased the bone mass of their spinal column by up to 5 per cent. This was in sharp contrast to another group of women who did no exercise at all. By contrast, the second group was found to have lost an extra 7 per cent of their starting spinal bone mass within the same period of time the others had gained bone density.

In addition, forms of exercise which condition and strengthen muscles (yoga, Pilates and weight training) give us a twofold advantage when it comes to protecting our bones. When we have strong muscles, our co-ordination and physical reflexes are likely to be greatly improved. This has the huge benefit of substantially lessening our risk of falls and accidents. Yoga is especially helpful within this context, since it encourages us to develop a keen sense of balance and co-ordination, as well as formidable muscular strength. Secondly, resilient, well-conditioned muscles can provide an extremely effective physical buffer if a fall does occur, giving us important padding that can cushion the impact on our bones.

As we have already seen in 'Mind over Matter' (Chapter 3), regular exercise plays an extremely important role in balancing adrenal gland and hormone function. Since the latter also includes sex hormones, we should regard regular exercise as a vital tool in helping us make the transition of menopause as smoothly and untraumatically as possible. If we are experiencing an overload of continuing stress, and are unaware of basic techniques for stress-reduction (see Chapter 2) we are at great risk of suffering from overworked and exhausted adrenal glands.

This can aggravate health problems at any stage in our lives, but burnt out adrenal glands have a particular significance for us as we approach and move through menopause. This is linked to the way that our adrenal glands produce oestronel (a form of oestrogen) and androgens (male hormones). We need the balancing action of adrenal gland secretions to create the hormonal 'buffer' that can help carry us through the transitional phase of menopause. If, on the other hand, our adrenal glands have been exhausted through years of constant stress, they are far from likely to be up to the job that is required of them.

Regular exercise, on the other hand, plays a centrally important role in any effective stress-reduction programme. As a result, it is one of our great allies in supporting effective adrenal gland functioning. When we engage in regular exercise that conditions our hearts and lungs, we provide an outlet for the excess adrenaline that goes coursing around our systems every time our bodies go on 'red alert' in response to a stressful trigger.

By burning off excess adrenaline in this way, we are effectively helping to reduce the pressure on our adrenal glands. If we also engage in forms of exercise that have a built-in relaxation component, we are also doing our adrenal glands a huge favour, and making it likely that they will not let us down when we need them most.

Exercise and heart health

When we consider how we can protect ourselves against developing heart and circulatory problems from mid-life onwards, we cannot overestimate the crucially important role played by aerobic exercise. If we only take one step towards looking after our hearts, getting physically fit should take top priority, since the rewards that come as a result of regular exercise are so considerable.

These benefits include greater efficiency of the heart in pumping blood around the body, and a slower resting pulse rate. The latter is significant because it is often regarded as a basic indicator of a well-functioning, healthy heart. Regular demands made through exercise can also increase the size of the heart. When this happens through getting fitter (as opposed to the way a heart can become unhealthily enlarged as a result of disease), it is considered an advantage. As the heart becomes bigger, it has the capacity to pump a larger volume of blood with each beat. The desirable consequence is that it is not required to beat as frequently in order to achieve the same result. This is why a slower resting pulse rate can be used as a basic indicator of heart health.

It helps if we remember that the heart is basically a muscle, and in common with other major muscles in our bodies, it must be worked if it is to stay in condition. We all know how the muscles in our upper arms and thighs look and feel if they are regularly worked out, and how quickly they lose condition if they are stubbornly neglected. Although we cannot see what is happening to our hearts, the same rules apply. By taking sensible action sooner rather than later, we can condition our hearts to work more efficiently, saving us from premature symptoms of breathlessness, tightness in the chest, and eventually chest pain on exertion.

Instead of waiting until we see the obvious signs of damage mentioned above, why not take preventive action as we approach mid-life? The best form of prevention involves taking up regular, enjoyable aerobic exercise which is one of the basic ways we can improve our cardiovascular performance (the functioning of our hearts and circulatory system). When we exercise aerobically we make our hearts pump harder in an effort to transport fresh, oxygenated blood to other muscles of the body.

If we are unfit, the golden rule of starting aerobic activity is moderation. For the best results, never launch into an ambitious programme that may be so unrealistic and taxing that it does more harm than good. Start slowly with a routine that involves no more than five minutes of heart conditioning activity (this could be something simple like walking or cycling on an exercise bike) every other day. Add on an extra five minutes of activity each week until the thirty-minute point is reached.

Don't feel that this regime has to be rigidly stuck to; always listen to your body while you are exercising, and only take on further challenges when you feel you are ready to. This may mean that you feel it's more appropriate for you to keep at the level of exercising for five minutes every other day for three or four weeks before you are ready to move on. Don't deliberately avoid challenges you are able to take, but don't tax your body beyond a point that feels appropriate either. If you move on at your own individually determined pace, you are far more likely to be successful in building an effective fitness programme.

Exercise and emotional well-being

Approaching menopause can be a strange and confusing phase of life when many of us may feel a tumult of conflicting emotions running through our minds. On the one hand, we are going to be aware that we have more self-knowledge than at any other time of our lives, and our confidence levels will have dramatically increased since our formative years. By the time mid-life approaches, we will be less easily thrown by challenging situations, because of the wealth of experience that we can draw on. As a result, we should feel more grounded and balanced during this phase than in any other previous decade.

However, there are insidious nagging doubts that can arise at this very time when we should be feeling in our prime. These are often related to fears about our bodies showing signs of ageing, and as a result, an overwhelming sense of panic about losing physical attractiveness, strength and sexual confidence. If we aren't vigilant, this is when depressive feelings can hit us hard which can make the situation much worse, by lowering our levels of self-esteem even further.

One of the most powerful ways of combating this unpleasant downward spiral is to be found in taking regular, pleasurable exercise. By engaging in a balanced range of exercise that we enjoy, we can make an enormous positive difference to how we feel about our bodies. After all, who isn't likely to feel more confident with a body that is stronger, leaner and more flexible through exercising?

More significantly, regular physical activity also has a powerful positive effect on our brain chemistry. This involves the secretion of chemicals called endorphins into our bloodstreams. These chemicals are naturally occurring antidepressants that are responsible for the emotional 'high' that we experience as a result of aerobic exercise. Apart from making us feel good, endorphins also have a calming, sedative effect. This is why taking regular exercise is an excellent way of combating feelings of mild to moderate anxiety and depression.

There are obvious benefits to becoming physically fitter in preference to popping a pill like a tranquilliser in order to suppress our symptoms temporarily. Instead of experiencing the side effects that inevitably come with taking medication, regular exercise brings positive advantages with it when we use it as a mood-balancing ally. These extremely desirable benefits include healthier heart and lung performance, enhanced energy levels, improved immune system functioning, as well as sounder sleep patterns.

Most important of all, taking exercise at mid-life provides us with a vitally important sense of taking control and making a positive difference to our bodies. This is especially significant since, approaching menopause, many of us feel that we are suddenly powerless in the face of physical change. Yes, change is inevitable, but it need not inevitably be a change for the worse. On the contrary, as we have seen in the previous sections of this book, we still have time at menopause to make vitally important changes in our lifestyle that can make us genuinely healthier and more balanced than we thought possible.

Getting moving: basic issues

Too many of us are put off exercising by being overly ambitious in our aims at the outset, with the inevitable result that we become quickly discouraged and give up. The basic secret of making a regular fitness programme part of our lives is to be ruthlessly realistic about the sort of commitment we know we can keep up. We may have an ideal image in our minds of going to the gym or going for a swim every day after work, but if we have a busy social life, or demanding professional commitments that can change at a moment's notice, this sort of approach just isn't going to work.

Above all else. make sure that you become aware of the best time of day for you to exercise. This is different for each of us: some are at their best first thing in the morning, others in the late afternoon, and still more in the evening. This is determined by what homoeopaths refer to as our individual constitutional make-up, and should never be ignored. After all, it is just another way of getting to know our bodies; something which is a basic requirement of any successful fitness programme.

Most of the following advice is basic common sense, but it is amazing how easy it is to forget the obvious when we want to do something ambitious.

- The most important consideration for us at the outset should be the fun factor. Without the spark of pleasure we are going to become incredibly inventive about all of the reasons we have for not exercising. And who could blame us if we feel bored to tears? Whatever fitness activities we choose must resonate with our individual temperaments and personalities, as well as our basic fitness level.
- Work within your fitness level to start with, becoming more ambitious as you gain strength, stamina and flexibility. If you are a beginner don't try to do too much at first, but concentrate instead on the areas that you feel need most attention, and slowly but steadily move on to other goals.
- Be ruthlessly realistic about the amount of time you can genuinely give to exercising with the intention of making it a long-term commitment. Always be realistic rather than overly ambitious, and you are likely to find that you will be able to keep your fitness regime going. In addition, once you have a stable routine established you will find that you become happy to devote extra time to your fitness programme, as you are seeing extra results. This is the best way for a more ambitious schedule to develop, since when it grows in an organic way it stands a much better chance of continuing. This is in sharp contrast to putting unrealistic demands on ourselves at the beginning that will almost certainly result in our giving up.
- If you have tried getting fit and failed in the past, it can be

helpful to consider how imaginative you may have been in your chosen exercise activities. This time be more consciously aware of what is likely to be enjoyable and deliberately choose a form of exercise that suits your personality. If you find an appropriate match you are far more likely to be successful in getting and keeping fit.

The following table gives an idea of the general benefits involved in each exercise activity. The more unfamiliar exercise systems (t'ai chi or Pilates) are described in the section following the table.

Type of activity	Basic benefits
Brisk walking or 'power' walking	Improves bone density Conditions the heart and lungs Increases energy Improves muscle strength Enhances ease of movement in joints
Swimming	Conditions the heart and lungs Strengthens muscles Increases strength and flexibility in the joints Increases energy
Dancing	Conditions the heart and lungs Improves muscle strength Increases flexibility co-ordination
Cycling	Conditions the heart and lungs Builds muscle strength Increases energy
Aqua aerobics	Builds stamina Improves muscle strength Conditions the heart and lungs

Type of activity	Basic benefits
The Alexander Technique	Increases flexibility Encourages a sense of body awareness Enhances ability for muscular relaxation Improves postural alignment
Body sculpting	Improves muscular strength and tone Increases flexibility in muscles and joints Improves stamina
Weight training	Improves muscular strength and stamina Improves bone density Increases flexibility in muscles and joints
Pilates	Improves muscular strength and flexibility Improves flexibility and strength of joints Enhances ability for muscular relaxation Improves postural alignment
Yoga	Improves energy levels Enhances muscular strength and flexibility Improves bone density Improves flexibility and strength of joints Enhances ability for muscular relaxation Improves postural alignment Promotes a greater sense of emotional and physical balance

Type of activity	Basic benefits
T'ai chi	Enhances muscular and emotional relaxation Improves co-ordination flexibility and strength of joints and muscles Improves postural alignment Increases energy levels
Jogging	Conditions the heart and lungs Improves bone density Increases energy levels
Racket games (badminton, tennis, etc.)	Improves bone density Enhances strength and flexibility of joints and muscles

The following gives us a rough idea of how much time we should devote to each activity when we get started.

Improving bone density

Build up consistently to three thirty-minute sessions of weight-bearing exercise a week. In addition, build as much weight-bearing activity into your daily routine as possible. This can be easily incorporated by walking rather than taking the car or bus for small trips.

Conditioning the heart and lungs

Try to aim for three thirty-minute sessions a week. Remember that in choosing to make walking your fitness activity you can look after bone density as well as your cardiovascular fitness level. In addition, make sure you take stairs rather than lifts and escalators whenever possible.

Improving flexibility

Start by aiming for fifteen-minute sessions two or three times a week. Slowly build up to thirty-five minutes' exercise which should ideally be done four or five times a week. When concentrating on exercises that promote muscular flexibility, it's important to allow one or two days that are exercise-free in order to allow your muscles to relax fully.

Enhanced muscle strength and muscle tone

Aim for three fifteen-minute sessions a week, building up to three thirty-minute sessions a week. Don't forget that most systems of exercise that improve muscle strength also help promote general flexibility. As a result, you can achieve both goals in the same half-hour session.

General muscular relaxation and stress reduction

Your chosen activity can be done whenever you feel generally tense and in need of relaxation. This could involve no more than five minutes spent doing a relaxing breathing exercise, or spending twenty to thirty minutes doing a full-scale relaxation technique.

Whole-body approaches to exercise

This section provides a quick introduction to some of the less obvious exercise systems mentioned above.

Yoga

The benefits of regular yoga practice cannot be overemphasised since it provides one of the most impressive body-conditioning systems available. When engaged in on a regular basis it appears to promote muscular suppleness, strength and balance, while also improving the functioning of the circulatory system. It can have a profound body-sculpting effect, while also helping to guard against osteoporosis. Yoga postures involve working the muscles hard enough to exert tension on the bones. It has been suggested that this pulling on the bones helps preserve bone density.

In addition, yoga postures involve building muscle strength and stamina as well as improving co-ordination. As a result of this greater sense of physical balance, there is a reduced risk of falling as a result of poor co-ordination. Even if a fall does occur, well-conditioned, strong muscles can provide an essential physical buffer that can help protect against fractures.

Yoga has also been hailed as one of the most effective anti-ageing systems of movement that we can engage in. This is partly due to the way that the postures regularly involve working against gravity by stretching, lengthening and elongating the muscles as much as possible. Since there is a central component of learning how to breathe from the diaphragm in yoga, it provides us with the additional benefit of increased oxygen absorption and effective stress reduction. As we have already seen, both of these factors are powerful allies if we want to avoid signs of premature ageing. In addition, it has been suggested that daily yoga practice may help regulate metabolism, balance the hormonal system, boost energy levels, focus the mind, and keep the spine supple and strong.

Yoga is likely to be a particularly attractive system of exercise for anyone who may have been alienated from the idea of exercise in their youth as a result of an overly tough or competitive atmosphere. Yoga will come as a breath of fresh air for anyone who feels this way, since in daily practice we are in competition with no one. We are encouraged to measure our progress with our own previous performance, and not in competition with anyone else. As a result, we should never be tempted to force our bodies beyond any boundary where we begin to feel under undue pressure or discomfort.

The system of yoga we are generally most familiar with in the West is called hatha yoga. This is a system of movement that empowers us to develop a finer sense of consciousness through initially developing the body. Hatha yoga focuses very much on developing physical qualities of strength and suppleness. This is achieved through the incorporation of demanding stretches and fluid movements that, when executed correctly, stimulate energy levels, improve muscle strength, stamina, flexibility and overall shape. Although challenging at first, regular practice of yoga can yield startling rewards in the form of an enhanced sense of confidence, vitality and well-being.

When initially learning the basics of yoga, it is extremely important to take a course of lessons from a trained teacher. Within the context of a well-taught class we will learn how to do basic postures and how to breathe from the diaphragm. This is of great importance, since there is a danger that, if we try to learn the basics at home, we will be doing the postures incorrectly. This leaves us open to injury at worst, and the risk of not gaining the potential benefits of yoga postures at best.

Once we are confident that we know the basics thoroughly, it can be helpful to supplement time spent in class with practice at home. Using a videotape (ideally try to get a recommendation from your teacher) can be very helpful. Your teacher may also recommend home practice and may produce a worksheet that you should follow.

Pilates

In common with yoga, Pilates (pronounced Pill-ah-tays) provides us with one of the most effective all-purpose, anti-ageing forms of exercise. It is a body conditioning system of movement initially developed by Joseph Pilates. These days it has become extremely popular, with increasing numbers of trainers teaching in workout studios or providing one-to-one personal training sessions.

The Pilates method of exercise lays great emphasis on the need for an acute sense of body awareness to develop while exercising. If this doesn't happen, maximum benefit is not likely to be gained from the very precise movements involved in this system of exercise.

Those of us who suffer from unconditioned, poorly toned muscles can benefit greatly from the Pilates approach. The beauty of this method is that although muscles are worked hard, the technique does not result in a 'muscle-bound' look. On the contrary, Pilates exercises will improve muscle tone by stretching tight, bunched-up muscles, and strengthening weak, flabby ones. As a result of improved muscle condition, our bodies should appear leaner and longer. We may also find that regular practice of Pilates will make us feel sleeker as a result of the greater consciousness of posture and alignment that this method brings.

In common with yoga, which is tailored to suit the needs and pace of development of each individual, Pilates will not force anyone into a position with which they feel uncomfortable or instinctively ill at ease. This is a system of exercise that can improve muscle strength, reduce stress, increase flexibility, and make us increasingly aware of negative postural habits we may have adopted over the years as a form of 'body armouring' against stressful or traumatic stimuli.

Successful practice of the Pilates method involves movements that work specific muscle groups in a very precise, conscious way for a limited number of repetitions. Since it is of paramount importance to learn how to do these movements correctly in order to gain maximum benefit from them, teaching is initially best given on an individual basis or within the context of a class of strictly limited number.

Because of this need for maximum accuracy, there is initially no substitute for learning the technique from an experienced teacher. Once the technique is mastered, home practice may be supplemented by using a home video tape ideally recommended by your teacher.

T'ai chi

In common with yoga, t'ai chi lays great emphasis on the need to breathe in a relaxed, conscious way. The combination of breathing techniques with slow, graceful movements to be found in t'ai chi practice is thought to stimulate and regulate the flow of vital energy (called chi) through the body. When t'ai chi is practised regularly it appears to balance energy levels, promote relaxation through relaxing the nervous system, increase co-ordination, and improve all-round flexibility. In addition, it encourages us to breathe to maximum efficiency while avoiding causing any undue strain on the heart.

Because the synchronisation of movements with breathing is so important, it is best to learn t'ai chi from a trained teacher. This gives us the maximum chance of getting to grips with the basic movements at our optimum pace. Within this context, any adjustments can be made by the teacher as and when the need arises. Classes can be given on a one-to-one basis. or in larger groups that can include anything up to twenty members.

The general atmosphere in a class should feel relaxed and unstressed, with a great deal of the emphasis being laid on breathing techniques. It is best to aim for daily practice if possible, with back up being given from a weekly taught class. As with yoga and Pilates, once we have mastered the basic techniques involved in t'ai chi, we can use video tapes at home to help us with our daily practice.

The Alexander Technique

Although the Alexander Technique is not an exercise system, it is an important technique to consider when we are discussing the subject of developing a sense of body-awareness. Those who can benefit from this treatment include anyone who has become uncomfortably aware of postural problems through recurrent bouts of neck, shoulder or joint pain. In addition, symptoms that have developed as a result of injury, or occupations that include repetitive movements (such as dancing or playing a musical instrument) appear to respond well to learning the Alexander Technique.

Perhaps most significantly of all, this technique has the major benefit of teaching us a great deal about how our emotions affect our posture and vice versa. As a result, once we have become attuned to the way in which we tense ourselves up in response to stress, we can choose to respond in a more relaxed way. Being given the chance to loosen ourselves up in this way can give us the opportunity of releasing energy that can otherwise be wasted in feeling stressed out and tense.

Learning the Alexander Technique can be particularly appropriate at times of great change and adjustment, since it can make us aware of the intimate links between our emotions and the way in which we hold our bodies. Once we can identify what these postural habits are, we are free to change emotional responses that we might previously have thought of as purely instinctive and ingrained.

We are empowered in doing this by becoming aware of how we react physically when we are faced with people or situations that we perceive as threatening or stressful. Once we are familiar with these physical reactions, we can learn a great deal about the negative aspects of these coping strategies. Once we can stand back from an emotional situation in this way, we can decide for ourselves if another way of responding might not be better for us.

This may all sound a little far-fetched at first, but take a moment next time you are aware of feelings of tension or slight depression, and bring your attention to the changes in your posture. When reacting to a stressful situation, almost all of us tighten up our muscles in a form of 'body armouring'. This often causes us to clench our jaws together, tighten the muscles of the face and neck, while tense shoulders are drawn up towards the ears. This has the further effect of making the upper and lower back rigid and tense, which can cause problems with tension headaches, and chronic neck and shoulder pain. Since holding our muscles in a state of tension in this way is very energy-consuming, there is a good chance that we will feel lethargic, sluggish and weary if we keep responding to stress in this way.

On the other hand, this is only one perspective on this situation, since we can choose to react differently once we know how to break a habitual response. Once we become more in tune with the reactions of our bodies under pressure we can change our postural reactions so that we feel less tense or anxious. So, if we can change our posture according to how we feel, we can also change how we feel by adjusting our posture.

Since we are trying to break habits that are likely to have been learnt since childhood, this process is unlikely to happen overnight. More to the point, a more aligned, balanced posture can initially feel strange and uncomfortable to us. The chances are that we will spend most of our time at first wanting to return to poor postural habits that feel more familiar, regardless of how many problems they may be causing.

Always remember that if we steadily develop a sense of awareness of our bodies, this can be a vital ally in helping us through episodes of emotional crisis, once we understand the signals our bodies are sending us. This is, in the long run, much more satisfactory than constantly bracing ourselves in a state of mental and emotional tension that can lead to a spiral of negative stress and exhaustion.

When learning the Alexander Technique there is little point in trying to teach ourselves with the help of a book, since if we do it incorrectly we are hardly likely to gain the maximum benefit. Try to locate a teacher trained in the technique who can give you lessons ideally on a one-to-one basis. You may be surprised at first to discover that a lot of time in class will be spent doing nothing more ambitious than sitting down and rising out of a chair. However, you are likely to be amazed at how much these simple movements can teach you about the way in which you use your body. Your teacher is also likely to make suggestions about ways you can practise the technique at home in order to make maximum progress between lessons.

6

The Medicated Menopause: the Pros and Cons of Hormone Replacement Therapy

Deciding whether or not to take hormone replacement therapy (HRT) is one of the biggest decisions we can make with regard to maximising and protecting our overall experience of health during and following the menopause. It really isn't too surprising that we may be unsure about which choice to make, especially if we haven't yet got to grips with the basic issues surrounding the conflicting opinions of conventional medical wisdom and an alternative medical approach. Orthodox doctors view the menopause in a specific way as a hormone deficiency problem, while alternative and complementary practitioners view it as a natural and inevitable transitional phase of life that requires maximum support in order to be accomplished as smoothly and in as positive a way as possible.

This chapter aims to put the basic arguments for and against HRT within a realistic and responsible context, so that the arguments for and against conventional and alternative treatment are made as accessible as possible. The information that follows does not claim to be a definitive, totally bang-up-to-the-minute survey, but it does aim to highlight the essential points that most of us will want to have access to in order to get closer to an informed and satisfying choice of treatment.

It may also be helpful to make it clear from the outset that what we are considering in this chapter is a broad spectrum of choices rather than a stark 'either/or' choice. As a practitioner I see some patients who are committed to continuing with HRT, who want additional positive support from a homoeopathic perspective, others, who are uneasy with HRT, who want homoeopathic treatment to help them make the transition away from HRT, while others feel totally uneasy with the concept of being treated with HRT and want to use only alternative medical means to support them through their problems with menopause.

Menopause from a conventional medical perspective

Conventional doctors will often refer to the menopause as an oestrogen deficiency state set in motion by the progressively dwindling amount of the hormone oestrogen being secreted by the ovaries in the years leading up to the menopause. By the time this transitional phase actually occurs, oestrogen levels will have dropped to a minimal level and progesterone secretion will have virtually ceased. Doctors acknowledge that not all women will go through a uniform experience as their hormone levels are changing, since the time of onset of the menopause, and severity and range of symptoms, can be influenced by a number of factors.

These may include body weight (women who are slightly above their recommended body weight will have greater oestrogen reserves in fatty tissues and as a result may suffer less severe oestrogen deficiency symptoms), surgical intervention that can provoke a premature menopause, and hereditary factors, including the menopausal symptoms experienced by close female relatives.

On the other hand, there are certain symptoms that can

predictably happen around the time of the menopause that are regarded from the conventional medical perspective as being linked to dwindling reserves of oestrogen. These may include a formidably wide range of physical, sexual or emotional problems, including any of the following:

- Altered nature of periods: too often, less frequent, too heavy, more painful, or extremely light.
- Vaginal dryness.
- Increased likelihood of developing recurrent infections including thrush and/or cystitis.
- Dryness of skin and hair due to loss of collagen which gives skin its supportive base and elasticity. It has been claimed that HRT may replace lost collagen within six months of initial use.
- Hot flushes, night sweats and palpitations.
- Adverse changes of bones and blood vessels (loss of strength and elasticity).
- Diminished libido.
- Painful intercourse.
- Mood swings including irritability, anxiety and depression.
- Memory loss.

Generally speaking, conventional doctors tend to divide menopausal problems into two categories: those that are of 'nuisance value' (hot flushes, night sweats, vaginal discomfort, mood swings, and loss of libido), and those that are potentially life-threatening and therefore extremely serious (coronary heart and circulatory disease and osteoporosis (loss of bone density)). It is the second category that most of the discussion relating to HRT tends to centre around. In other words, HRT is recommended as a useful option for easing the distressing symptoms of hot flushes, but it is portrayed as being essential in providing protection against the more serious problems of osteoporosis and heart disease.

The conventional view and treatment of osteoporosis

In order to help us understand the conventional treatment for osteoporosis, we need to grasp the basic facts about how and when bone density is formed and maintained. Bone is essentially made up of a form of connective tissue which reaches its maximum density in women at around thirty-five years of age. Bony tissue is composed of approximately one-third of collagen (which contributes strength and elasticity) and two-thirds of mineral content. The latter is primarily composed of the mineral calcium: it is primarily the loss of this constituent of bone which leads to problems with brittleness and easy fracturing when it begins to leach away in the menopausal and post-menopausal years.

It is important to bear in mind that bony tissue is not something that is static in nature and composition, but it is constantly being modified in its nature by the opposing action of cells called osteoblasts and osteoclasts. In optimum conditions, these cells work in a balanced way, with osteoblasts building up bony tissue and osteoclasts breaking down, or encouraging the reabsorption of cells that are surplus to requirements. The delicate balance between these two essential processes for promoting and maintaining healthy, resilient bones is governed by the smooth and harmonious functioning of a range of hormone and growth factors including the oestrogen and progesterone. Within this context, oestrogen prevents reabsorption of bone while progesterone initiates bone formation.

The basic background to osteoporosis

Once the ovaries fail to function and excessive amounts of bone calcium begin to be excreted from the body as a result of lowered levels of oestrogen and progesterone secretion, bone mass is generally compromised, as well as collagen and mineral levels being adversely affected. While this will generally happen to women over the age of sixty in varying degrees of severity, there are certain predictable factors that can make osteoporosis more likely to occur at an earlier age, or in a more severe form. These include any of the following:

- An absence of periods due to a hormone imbalance with too much prolactin circulating in the bloodstream.
- Lack of periods due to a history of eating disorders and/or an excessively low body weight as a result of strenuous physical exercise (dancers and athletes are especially at risk).
- An early menopause (before the age of forty-five) which can happen naturally, as the result of surgery, or treatment for cancer with chemotherapy and/or radiotherapy.
- A history of severe osteoporosis in close female relatives.
- Having a compact build with small frame and fine, short bones.
- Cigarette smoking.
- High or regular alcohol intake.
- No pregnancies.
- A sedentary lifestyle.
- A history of bone disease before the menopause has set in.
- High caffeine intake (from fizzy drinks and tea as well as coffee).
- Using thyroxine (to treat an under-active thyroid gland) or steroids (often used to ease symptoms of asthma or rheumatoid arthritis and other auto-immune diseases).
- Asian and Caucasian women are thought to be more at risk of developing osteoporosis than African women.

General preventive measures

It has been acknowledged, bearing in mind the information given in the list above, that there are specific changes in lifestyle that can be made in order to protect against osteoporosis setting in at an early phase, and in a severe way. These include the following:

- Dietary protection should begin as early as possible (especially important if we consider that maximum bone density has been established by our mid-thirties). Daily intake of food should

119

be as balanced and nutritious as possible, including regular supplies of vitamin D, calcium and magnesium.

- Alcohol intake should be kept within strictly moderate limits (well within the weekly recommended limit for women of fourteen units).

- Regular weight-bearing exercise is a must in any osteoporosis prevention programme, since it appears to discourage excessive leaching of calcium from the large bones in the hip and thighs. For optimum results, aim for twenty to thirty minutes of weight-bearing exercise four times a week. Excellent types of physical activity include brisk walking, jogging (ideally on a soft, springy surface in order to minimise sharp, jolting movements that put excessive pressure on joints), tennis and aerobic dancing. Weight-bearing exercise has a double-edged positive effect, since its benefits are not limited to discouraging de-mineralisation of bone but, in addition, it also improves overall muscle tone and balance. As a result, there is likely to be a reduced risk of fractures that can happen as a direct result of falls resulting from poor co-ordination.

- Caffeine intake should be drastically cut down or eliminated, and smokers should make every effort possible to give up the habit since both factors have been shown to contribute to problems with osteoporosis.

- Convenience foods containing high proportions of phosphorus should be eliminated from the diet, since too much phosphorus has an adverse effect on absorption of calcium from the diet. Foods to avoid for this reason include canned or otherwise preserved meats, instant soups and fizzy drinks.

However, the major weapon that conventional medicine believes it has in its armoury when fighting osteoporosis is HRT. Women who are considered especially vulnerable to developing the condition because they have a high proportion of the risk factors mentioned above, or who have experienced easy fractures of the wrist, are likely to be advised to use HRT in order to protect against further loss of bone density.

The thinking behind this approach, put extremely simply, is

that because loss of bone density accelerates in the post-menopausal years, this must be linked to dropping oestrogen levels. The solution from a conventional perspective is straightforward: boost flagging oestrogen levels by supplementing with HRT, since oestrogen has been shown to encourage the uptake of calcium from the blood into bony tissue, and can inhibit leaching from the bones.

In addition, menopausal symptoms that are also associated with dwindling oestrogen reserves from a conventional medical perspective (hot flushes, night sweats, thinning of the walls of the vagina, and lowered libido) are also regarded as benefiting from a booster supply of oestrogen through the use of HRT.

Heart health and HRT

The second serious problem that can arise for women in the years following the menopause is an elevated risk of developing cardiovascular disease. When women are in their thirties, the risk of their developing heart disease is six times lower than men in the same age group. However, by the time they reach their seventies, the incidence of heart disease is virtually the same for both men and women. The conventional medical explanation for this change in pattern for women, once they are well past the menopause, is linked to changes that take place in blood-clotting factors and arteries at this time. According to *The Which? Guide: Understanding the Menopause*, a number of studies have suggested that ovarian sex hormones play an important role in protecting women from developing coronary heart disease. This appears to be linked to the way that oestrogen has a widening effect on the smooth muscle of artery walls, thus promoting an improved volume of blood flow.

Recent opinion also suggests that female body shape and distribution of body fat may also play a relevant part in predicting whether we are at a higher risk of developing cardiovascular disease or not. The classic male-type distribution of body fat over the upper body and belly may signify a negative profile with greater risk of circulatory disease, while fat deposits that settle more on the lower half of the body on the hips and thighs may suggest a reduced risk of developing coronary heart disease. Within this overall context, the claim has been made that use of HRT may reduce the tendency to develop the former male-type pattern in favour of the latter.

However, it is important to point out that the role that HRT may play in a preventive capacity against developing heart disease is a very controversial issue. Some sources suggest that these are far too early days to draw hard and fast conclusions, since some of the studies have shown alarmingly contradictory results. For instance, 27,000 women taking part in an HRT trial in the United States were recently sent letters warning of a possible increased risk of heart attack. Worries had surfaced during the American trial when it emerged that the number of women suffering from a heart attack, stroke, or blood clot was above average.

Additional factors that point to a potentially elevated risk of heart disease may include a combination of any of the following:

* A history of high blood pressure.
* Naturally occurring or surgically induced premature menopause.
* Diabetes.
* Smoking.
* Being overweight.
* A sedentary lifestyle.
* A poor diet that is high in a combination of saturated fat and sugar.
* High stress levels.

General preventive measures

* Regular, gentle, appropriate exercise that is tailored to a realistic level of fitness is of vital importance in encouraging heart health as well as discouraging osteoporosis if it's of a weight-bearing nature.
* The overall nature of the diet should be nutritious and well

balanced in order to encourage maintenance of an optimum weight. Generally speaking, dietary guidelines for a healthy heart should also encourage a healthy weight: high in fibre, low in sugar, no more than 20 per cent of dietary fat, moderate alcohol, and high in complex carbohydrates.

- Alcohol should be kept well within the weekly recommended amount: ideally no more than a glass of red wine each day.
- Above all else, smoking should be avoided because of its generally negative effect in promoting cardiovascular disease as well as its controversial relationship to lung cancer.

Using hormone replacement therapy

Hormone replacement therapy was first used in the 1950s, in the form of oestrogen replacement therapy in United States, as a treatment for dwindling oestrogen reserves in those women struggling with menopausal symptoms. Unfortunately, it became apparent that were serious problems associated with the oestrogen-only formula that was being given, since its use led to an unacceptably high risk of developing cancer of the lining of the womb (estimated as a tenfold risk after ten to fifteen years of use).

To combat this tendency, a synthetic form of progesterone called progestogen was added to HRT formulas by the 1960s as a way of discouraging the thickening of womb-lining that could too often be the precursor of endometrial cancer. This has also been found to have certain disadvantages of its own, since the action of progestogen appears to negate the potentially positive effect that oestrogen may have on blood lipid levels. As a result, it is unlikely to have a positive role to play in helping to protect against coronary heart disease.

Although we speak of HRT as though it is one thing, it is important to realise that the method of administration, dosage and combination of formulas vary greatly. This is partly why so many issues surrounding HRT can seem contradictory or downright confusing.

Types

HRT can be used in tablet, patch, gel, implant, vaginal cream or pessary form. Although in theory any of these routes of administration can be used, in practice the most commonly used method of delivering HRT in the UK and US is in tablet form. In France, however, HRT is far more likely to be used in the form of a gel called Oestogel which is applied to the arms, shoulders, and inner thighs. Although this method of delivering HRT is thought to relieve hot flushes and genito-urinary problems, its role in providing protection against coronary heart disease and osteoporosis is in question. There can also be drawbacks in the form of localised irritation and reddening of the skin (this can also occur when using patches), as well as a potential adverse reaction with detergents, cleansers, and skin-care products.

Although reactions to HRT may differ depending on the route of administration used, the following are the most commonly reported side effects:

- Bleeding
- Depression
- Breast tenderness
- PMS-type symptoms
- Irritation of the skin
- Weight gain
- Headaches

It is also important to bear in mind that there are certain conditions which can make the use of HRT inadvisable. These include any of the following:

- Diabetes
- Benign breast lumps
- Gall bladder disease
- Endometriosis
- Fibroids
- A history of inflamed varicose veins

- Liver disease
- A history of deep vein thrombosis or pulmonary embolism (blood clot in the lungs)
- A history of cancer of the breast or cancer of the womb

Authors such as Kitty Campion have also drawn attention to worrying statistics that suggest we may be substantially raising our risk of developing cancer of the breast or lining of the womb by using HRT if this is for more than ten years. A study conducted in 1995 revealed that women exposed to unopposed oestrogen had a seven times greater risk of developing cancer of the lining of the womb. It has also been suggested that HRT taken for more than ten years may also increase the risk of developing cancer of the ovaries by 70 per cent, according to an American study conducted in 1995.

Apart from undesirable side effects and contraindications, there are other, more general issues to consider that can make the use of HRT unappealing. One of the main disadvantages of using a combination of oestrogen and progestogen is that whatever a woman's age, she will continue to have a monthly bleed. For women in their sixties and beyond, this is likely to feel inappropriate and unappealing. It may also be one of the primary reasons why there is a poor track record in the UK for continued use of HRT. There are additional, more general psychological issues attached to the use of HRT that are discussed later in this chapter (see pp. 134–6).

Menopause from an alternative medical perspective

As we have pointed out at the start of this chapter, it can be extremely illuminating to realise that we do not have to make a simple choice between opting for conventional HRT or nothing. In fact, there are a number of options open to us for managing our transition through menopause that may or may not include using supplementary hormones. These include seeking alternative medical treatment from homoeopaths, herbalists or nutritionists, and/or considering using progesterone cream.

At the heart of any form of alternative medical approach lies the concept that each of us is an individual who experiences health and ill health in her own unique way. In other words, while there may be common symptoms associated with menopause, each woman may differ in the severity and time of onset of her symptoms, and the same may be true with regard to her response to treatment.

Some of us may respond very positively to a nutritional and exercise programme alone, while others may find that they need extra help from herbal supplements or homoeopathic remedies. Some of us may have a history that suggests we may be at high risk of developing osteoporosis, while others may be more concerned about the possibility of heart disease. If these two issues are of major concern to us, them we may benefit from screening procedures in order to establish just how much at risk we are before we experience menopause. If we need extra therapeutic help we might investigate using progesterone cream.

However, the most important distinction of all between conventional and alternative medical perspectives is that while conventional doctors regard menopause as an illness in the form of an oestrogen deficiency state, alternative practitioners have a contrasting view of menopause as a major transitional life event. As a result, instead of providing treatment for an illness, most alternative practitioners regard their function as providing whatever support is needed to enable each woman to accomplish her passage through menopause as swiftly and successfully as possible. In providing this support, as much attention is likely to paid to emotional and psychological well-being as to physical symptoms.

The natural progesterone debate

Although not, strictly speaking, an 'alternative' treatment in the form of a traditional alternative or complementary therapy, the use of natural progesterone cream in supporting women through a difficult passage of menopause has generated great interest over recent years. Natural progesterone cream is synthesised in the laboratory from a plant source called wild yam. The hormone that is the end product is said to be identical to the progesterone produced by the body, unlike the synthetic form of progesterone (called progestogen) that is used in the contraceptive pill and conventional HRT.

Unlike conventional medical theory which regards menopausal symptoms as being related specifically to falling levels of oestrogen which must be boosted through HRT, pioneers of the use of progesterone cream, such as Dr John Lee in the United States, see menopausal problems as being linked to dramatically falling progesterone levels in the post-menopausal years.

Lee suggests that the argument in favour of supplementing oestrogen levels with synthetic oestrogens may well be aggravating an existing situation of hormone imbalance for women. In such a situation, oestrogen dominance can lead to a range of distressing symptoms including any of the following:

- Acceleration of the ageing process
- Allergic problems
- Breast tenderness
- Thickening of the lining of the womb
- Anxiety and depression
- Weight gain
- Fatigue
- Gall bladder disease
- Headaches and migraines
- Mood swings
- Fibroids
- Water retention
- Osteoporosis

Causes of oestrogen dominance

The argument in favour of oestrogen dominance suggests that we are constantly bombarded by synthetic oestrogens (called xenoestrogens) in our environment. Contact with any of the following may contribute to a situation of oestrogen dominance: pesticides, plastics, meat (injected with hormones, antibiotics, growth enhancers, etc.), soaps, exhaust fumes, the contraceptive pill, and oestrogen-only HRT.

Practical steps that we can take to limit our exposure to xenoestrogens may include any of the following:

- Decrease use of pesticides, garden sprays and house sprays wherever possible, trying to find organic, eco-friendly, alternatives.
- Eliminate foods from the diet that are most likely to be contaminated with these chemicals: meat, milk and coffee. Opt instead for organic substitutes that are free from hormone and antibiotic residues wherever possible.
- Wherever possible avoid exposure to solvents, plastics, cosmetics and soaps manufactured with petrochemical emulsifiers and spreaders.
- When choosing flooring materials, opt for natural wood or stone rather than carpet. The problem with the latter lies in the glues and solvents which attach the backing to the carpet – these can give off toxic molecules for years.
- Avoid use of synthetic hormones.

A question of balance: the nature of oestrogen dominance

When our hormone levels are working in a balanced way through our fertile years, our bodies produce oestrogen in the first half of our menstrual cycles, and this is balanced by the secretion of progesterone in the second half. Provided we ovulate each month, progesterone levels are produced that protect us against symptoms of progesterone deficiency, which may include swollen, painful breasts, cramps, weight gain, and mood swings. When our hormones work in a balanced, harmonious way we should find that PMS is not a problem, and the first indication we have that our period is due should be when the bleeding starts.

However, this is sadly far from the reality that many of us may experience if our hormones are in disarray. A wide variety of factors can influence our hormonal balance including thyroid imbalances, poor nutrition, taking conventional medication, and emotional stress. When our overall hormone balance is humming along nicely we feel energised, well, and in command, but when this delicate balance is upset we are vulnerable to respiratory problems, heart disease, cancer and osteoporosis. It is Dr Lee's opinion that one of the most powerful contributory factors in upsetting our hormonal balance is using the contraceptive pill during our fertile years, followed by years spent taking synthetic HRT during and following the menopause.

Oestrogen dominance is thought to occur where there may be low, normal, or excessive amounts of oestrogen, but little or no progesterone to balance its effect on the body. If we take on board that the fall of progesterone at menopause is proportionally much higher than the fall in oestrogen (oestrogen falls by approximately 40 to 60 per cent from baseline levels while progesterone levels fall to nearly zero), the scene may be easily set for oestrogen dominance to occur at this time.

Dr Lee does not dispute that genuine cases of oestrogen deficiency may occur, but suggests that some cases of oestrogen dominance may be mistaken for oestrogen deficiency. True symptoms of low oestrogen levels may be hot flushes, night sweats and vaginal dryness, which may be eased by using natural oestrogens to be found from plant sources. However, fatigue, impaired memory and muzzy-headedness may be due as much to oestrogen dominance as deficiency. When this mistake is made, and synthetic oestrogen is given, it can obviously aggravate an already unhappy situation.

Natural progesterone and osteoporosis and heart disease

It has been suggested that the use of natural progesterone cream combined with nutritional advice and an appropriate exercise programme may not only stop bone loss, but may actually reverse it. This is in contrast to conventional forms of HRT which appear to stop further bone loss once treatment begins, but which do not appear to be able to reverse the damage that may have already have been done. Both HRT and natural progesterone cream need to be taken on a long-term basis in order to maximise protection against osteoporosis. It has also been suggested that natural progesterone may have a normalising effect on blood-clotting factors and may reduce sodium and fluid retention. As a result, it may play a positive role in the prevention of thrombosis and high blood pressure, thus benefiting the circulatory system as a whole.

The most appropriate route of administration for progesterone cream is application to the skin on the palms of the hands, upper chest, wrists and neck where it is absorbed into fatty tissue before passing into the bloodstream.

Opinion is still divided about the use of progesterone cream, with a number of conventional doctors suggesting that not enough work has been done to support the use of natural progesterone for the relief of menopausal symptoms. Some alternative therapists and nutritionists have also suggested that the use of progesterone, however natural its molecular structure may be in relation to the body's own progesterone, is still a form of synthetic hormone replacement therapy. In other words, we may be repeating the same mistakes with supplementary progesterone that were made thirty years ago with oestrogen. There is also the persuasive argument that advocates of progesterone therapy are still working from the premise that menopause is a deficiency state rather than part of a natural process in a mature woman's life experience. Either way, it would seem that we need more time and evidence to be presented before we can be sure that there are few long-term problems associated with the use of natural progesterone.

Alternative routes of support: herbal and homoeopathic medicines

If menopausal symptoms are problematic, it is extremely helpful to discover that we have the potential for effective treatment at our disposal beyond the first resort of conventional HRT. Hot flushes, night sweats, recurrent urinary infections and dry vaginal tissues may respond very well to herbal or homoeopathic prescribing. See the 'Alternative Self-Help' section (Chapter 7) for a run-down of possible options of treatment.

Whether to choose herbal or homoeopathic treatment often depends on the practical issue of availability of treatment locally. In other words, if we have heard that there is an excellent herbalist practising nearby who has a great deal of expertise in treating women with menopausal problems this is likely to be an excellent place to start. If after a while sufficient progress isn't being made, then it would be worth exploring homoeopathic treatment. After all, it can't be emphasised enough that alternative practitioners treat each person as being unique in their individuality. As a result, what may work beautifully for one may not be appropriate for another.

It is important to stress that when alternative treatment is effective, a broad-based improvement should be seen rather than a piecemeal easing of some symptoms with other problems still being persistent. In other words, when alternative treatment is genuinely successful there should be a perceptible improvement right across the board, with an increased sense of emotional, mental and physical well-being. This is especially relevant to the treatment of menopausal conditions, since there is often a large component of energy loss and emotional distress accompanying physical symptoms such as hot flushes.

Alternative treatment has the additional advantage of a minimal risk of side effects from treatment. Unlike the conventional medical approach, which tends to use medicines which have a suppressive effect on the body (such as anti-inflammatories which will dampen down inflammation for a while, or antacids which have the same effect on stomach acid), alternative medicines such as homoeopathic remedies appear to act by supporting the body to resolve the problem itself. This has a particular bearing with regard to HRT, since many women find that once they stop taking it their hot flushes which were effectively suppressed for a while come back with a vengeance. The same is true of the use of

HRT for the treatment of osteoporosis, since once medication is stopped, bone loss begins once again.

It is also helpful to know that many alternative practitioners will be extremely informative about broader issues of lifestyle that can have a bearing on matters of concern such as heart disease and osteoporosis.

Effective strategies for deciding on an appropriate course of treatment for menopausal problems

If we are concerned about what treatment we need to consider in order to give ourselves maximum protection against problems developing as we move through menopause, the information that follows may put the choices open to us in a helpful, positive context.

- If symptoms have not yet materialised, but you are concerned about the possibility of osteoporosis developing, take a look at the section above entitled 'The basic background to osteoporosis' (pp. 118–21). If none or very few of the risk factors apply to you, and you have had no experience of easy fractures, you will benefit from taking on board the advice included in this section under the heading 'General preventive measures' (pp. 119–21). The same principles apply to concerns about heart and circulatory disease, since taking preventive steps with regard to relevant lifestyle changes can be enough to help us avoid unnecessary medical complications further down the line.
- If symptoms have arisen that may be linked to dwindling oestrogen levels such as hot flushes or night sweats, it is well worth considering alternative medical treatment as your first resort. See the chapter entitled 'Alternative Self-Help' (p. 137) for a run-down of appropriate options in treating common menopausal problems.
- Should persistent weight gain, mood swings, sluggishness, chilliness, or dizziness emerge during menopause, ask your GP

to do a blood test in order to check that thyroid function and iron levels are as they should be. Some of these symptoms can overlap with common features of menopause, and may be effectively identified and treated on their own merit without resorting to HRT.

- Those of us who may feel extremely vulnerable with regard to developing osteoporosis because of a high scoring on the potential list of risk factors (for example, early menopause through hysterectomy, strong family history of advanced osteo-porosis in close female relatives, or long-term use of steroids), should make it a priority to find out the base-line bone density we are working from as soon as possible. This can be done by arranging for a bone density scan to be done through your family doctor in order to establish in as objective a way as possible how much you may be at risk of genuine problems. If there are slight early signs of potential problems, making positive changes with regard to diet and exercise may be enough to address the situation. If further monitoring suggests that this may not be enough, professional treatment from a herbal, traditional Chinese or homoeopathic practitioner may provide the extra boost that is needed in order to stabilise the situation. If progesterone levels are revealed to be extremely low, it may also be worth considering the use of natural progesterone cream while continuing to have bone density assessed.

- If the choice is made to go ahead with conventional HRT it is also important to point out that this need not rule out additional options. These may include working out with the help of your consultant or general practitioner how to take the lowest dose of hormones in order to avoid side effects wherever possible, making sure that you avoid taking oestrogen-only preparations (see Dr John Lee for arguments in favour of always avoiding unopposed oestrogen), and making sure that relevant changes in lifestyle are not ignored. In addition, it is worth considering the use of any of the alternative therapies men-tioned above in order to give additional support to the body at this crucial time of transition. As a practitioner, I am aware that it may not be ideal to use homoeopathic treatment side by side with conventional medication, but the reality of life some-times involves situations that are less than perfect. As a result, it is not uncommon for practitioners to attempt treatment while their patient is receiving conventional medication, and it still appears to be valuable. This can be extremely liberating news for anyone who has previously made the decision to opt for HRT, who now feels that she would very much like to explore the benefits of an appropriate therapy, but thinks that this option was closed off to her as a result of a hastily made decision some time ago.

- Anyone who feels they may be at high risk of developing heart disease (see the risk factors listed in the 'Heart health and HRT' section on pp. 121–3) should take preventive steps as soon as possible. These involve straightforward and accessible lifestyle changes listed in the same section under the heading of 'General preventive measures' (pp. 122–3). It may also be helpful to have a few simple tests done in order to check that blood pressure is fine, and that cholesterol and blood sugar levels are within reasonable limits. Consulting an alternative practitioner (see therapies suggested above for prevention and treatment of slight osteoporosis) can also be an invaluable way of stimulating increased health and vitality right across the board, while also often providing an excellent source of additional advice on nutrition, exercise and relaxation.

The broader picture: deeper questions related to the use of HRT

In any discussion about the merits and demerits of using HRT, it is extremely important to move beyond a simple discussion of side effects and medical contraindications and consider the broader context of experiencing menopause. In order to do this effectively we need to stop for a while and think about the psychological effect of taking HRT, something that is rarely done in any conventional medical discussion about the menopause.

As we can see from the information given above, conventional doctors regard the menopause rather like any other illness that involves a deficiency state, such as diabetes. In other words, HRT is prescribed in order to rectify dwindling levels of oestrogen in much the same way that insulin-dependent diabetics rely on their doses of medication in order to keep blood sugar levels stable. However, there is a major difference that is overlooked whenever an analogy of this kind is made: diabetes is a genuine illness that does not occur when anyone is in good health and their bodies are functioning at their optimum level. Menopause, on the other hand, is not only inevitable after a predictable age, but like puberty, it is a major rite of passage rather than a disease state.

The situation is made even more complicated by the 'hype' and general claims made about the use of HRT promoted by the media. Many eminent, successful women have given us the impression that HRT is a must for keeping us youthful, sexy, energised and attractive, as well as protecting us against the dreaded diseases of osteoporosis and circulatory problems. While it is certainly true that a proportion of women may feel very positively about HRT and be reluctant to consider other options, there are many more who have felt let down and bitterly disappointed when they did not find it to be the elixir of youth that they were promised. After all, how could a form of medicine relieve emotional and physical problems associated with menopause if deeper issues relating to changing identity are not addressed?

Perhaps most important of all, it is interesting to consider that using HRT will not encourage us to embrace the concept of moving on to another stage of our lives, but is more inclined to keep us in a chemically induced state of 'freeze frame'. After all, who is really excited at the idea of having monthly bleeds after the age of sixty? This sense of things being on temporary 'hold' is also true with regard to the benefits of HRT, since once we stop taking it, many of the symptoms, such as hot flushes, may return. The claimed improvements in bone density can also be temporary since, once HRT is stopped, bone density will return to the state it was in before treatment was begun.

It is arguable that the whole ethos of treatment with HRT

involves a denial or suppression of the reality of menopause, with the result that we are discouraged from moving onwards and encouraged to hold on to our youth in an unrealistic way. The result is all too often a powerful sense of conflict and dissatisfaction, with the added problem that when we stop using HRT these issues are waiting in the wings ready to confront us with renewed force, often causing more havoc later that they would have done if they were confronted years before.

On the other hand, if we use the transitional phase of the menopause as a time when we learn how to become in tune with our bodies so that we can improve our overall health by eating well, taking appropriate exercise, and using alternative or complementary medicine to speed us through the transitional phase as smoothly as possible and with the minimum of side effects, we are likely to face the future with an increased sense of confidence and self-awareness.

7

Alternative Self-Help for Short-Term Symptoms

We have learned so far about all of the fundamental strategies we can use in order to make the transition through menopause as trouble-free as a possible. However, some of us may find that we still have some degree of problem with symptoms that we would rather not treat with conventional drugs. The good news is that the following common menopausal problems can be greatly relieved by using simple alternative medical measures combined with appropriate changes in lifestyle. Once we know how to support ourselves through these symptoms of transition we can feel empowered and strengthened, rather than lost and helpless.

If for any reason the following self-help measures do not prove effective enough, or if there is a perceptible improvement that keeps relapsing, don't be tempted to give up on the idea that alternative measures can help. It may be that your problems are more deep-seated, and as a result require medical assessment and management from a trained practitioner.

Hot flushes

It has been estimated that approximately 80 per cent of women can expect to experience some degree of hot flushing in association with the menopause. The intensity of flushes can vary enormously, with some of us having no more than the odd sensation of feeling overheated and slightly sweaty, while others find hot flushes a physical and psychological torture that is dreaded each time the early signs appear.

Symptoms of hot flushes can include any of the following:

- A vague sense of uneasiness or foreboding that something unpleasant is about to happen.
- A hot sensation that may move downward from the face and head, or from the waist and chest upwards.
- During a flush the skin may take on a flushed and bright red appearance, or there may be a sense of burning up inside without any obvious change in skin colour.
- Drenching sweats may follow hard on the heels of a flush, with the face, scalp and the breasts being especially affected.
- There may be a sense of exhaustion or being 'spaced out' and disoriented after a flush.

Flushes can set in out of the blue for no obvious reason, but there are specific triggers that may make flushes more likely to happen. These can include:

- Being in a pressured situation where there is a sense of feeling the focus of unwelcome attention.
- Surroundings that are overly warm or lacking in fresh air.
- Eating hot or spicy foods or drinking very hot liquids.
- Wearing synthetic fibres that do not allow the body to breathe and cool off quickly.

One of the factors that may make us more disposed to severe hot flushes may be the abruptness with which our supplies of the hormone oestrogen decrease and ovulation ceases. If this is a fairly gradual process, with slow but steady changes being reflected in the pattern of our periods, we stand a fighting chance that the severity of symptoms such as hot flushes may be minimal. On the other hand, if this process is much more erratic and unpredictable, problems with hot flushes may be correspondingly more severe.

Quick-fix hints

- Opt for layers of clothes rather than one warm garment, so that what you are wearing can be quickly adjusted to match your body temperature. If we bear in mind that hot flushes occur as a result of our body's in-built thermostat going haywire during the menopause, it makes a great deal of sense to dress in a way that allows us to respond to internal temperature change as quickly as possible. The best fabrics to choose include natural fibres that allow the skin to breathe such as linen, cotton or silk. Above all avoid synthetic fabrics such as microfibres that can contribute to feeling hot and bothered.
- Avoid foods and drinks that have a reputation for bringing on, or making hot flushes more severe or protracted. These include strong tea, coffee, alcohol, chocolate, sweetened or caffeinated drinks such as colas, and spicy dishes such as chillies or very hot curries. Opt instead for calming herbal teas or cool alcohol-free herbal drinks, and eat as many whole foods as possible such as pulses, raw fruit, raw vegetables, soya products and whole grains. If your diet has been pretty poor due to a recent period of stress or upheaval, consider supplementing with vitamins B complex, C and E for a limited period of time.
- If feelings of panic or anxiety are associated with hot flushes, it is well worth considering learning relaxation techniques or how to meditate. These can be practised at home with the minimum amount of fuss once the basic techniques have been learned from an audio or video tape.
- Becoming physically fit can do a great deal to help ease the symptoms of hot flushes. The most beneficial form of exercise to choose from is one that stimulates the circulatory system, but it must also be an activity that you enjoy or there is little

chance that you will continue. Possible options include brisk walking, tennis, swimming or dancing.

• Eating patterns can also have an impact on hot flushes, since low blood sugar (hypoglycaemia) can make symptoms worse. Keep blood sugar levels stable by making sure that small amounts of food are eaten every couple of hours, rather than allowing long gaps between meals and then making up for it by eating a large amount. Also avoid foods that have a reputation for giving a sugar 'rush' such as sweet, fizzy drinks, coffee, chocolate, or any items that are high in refined sugar.

Aromatherapy hints

A soothing and refreshing bath may be made by adding three drops of the following to warm water: *roman camomile, lavender* and/or *geranium*.

Homoeopathic hints

• Flushes that are made much worse by tight clothing around the neck and/or waist, and over-heated rooms, may respond to *lachesis*. Choice of this remedy would be confirmed by flushes being especially severe on waking from sleep, and severe mood swings that shift rapidly from depression to euphoria. This remedy would be worth considering if there is a past history of pre-menstrual syndrome.

• A general sensitivity to heat that occurs during menopause, if accompanied by an awful sense of becoming uncomfortably hot in bed at night, may require *sulphur*. A characteristic symptom that confirms choice of this remedy is the compulsion to push the feet outside the bedcovers at night in a desperate effort to cool down. Flushes may be much worse during, or following bathing, and may come on when standing for a long period of time.

• Upward moving flushes that are associated with a feeling of pressure in the head with dizziness and nausea may be relieved with a few doses of *glonoin*. Choice of this remedy would be confirmed if anxiety and palpitations occur with hot flushes as well as a very unpleasant sensation of disorientation.

- Hot flushes that come on when eating hot food or drinking hot drinks may respond to a few doses of *phosphorus*. Anxiety may accompany feeling flushes, with the whole body feeling as though it has been dipped in very hot water. Hot sweats may be especially marked on the head and hands.

Herbal hints

- Hot flushes that are linked to a state of 'burn-out' and general anxious exhaustion may respond to a course of oriental *ginseng* as an all-round tonic.
- Flushes may be eased by drinking an infusion of *sage* and *motherwort* which appear to contain oestrogen-like substances. A teaspoonful of each may be added to a cup of boiling water and left to stand before straining and drinking a tablespoon of the cooled mixture up to eight times a day. However, always bear in mind that *sage* shouldn't be used for more than a maximum of a week or two at a time, because of the potentially toxic effects of the volatile oil thujone that it contains.
- Oestrogen-like substances are also thought to be present in *dong quai* and *black cohosh* that can ease the misery of severe hot flushes. The latter is rich in phytosterols that allow hormone levels to re-balance themselves, and as a result can ease hot flushes as well as improving the whole system's ability to deal with stress. It can be taken in tincture form or as an infusion of the dried root, but it is important to bear in mind that it should never be used during pregnancy or where there is a marked tendency to menstrual flooding. *Dong quai*, on the other hand, can be extremely helpful where hot flushes emerge in anyone who is normally chilly by nature. This plant also has a reputation for thickening and moistening the tissues of the vagina, while also easing the symptoms of insomnia that can occur during the menopause. It can be taken in tincture or infusion of dried, powdered root, but it should be avoided if heavy periods, diarrhoea or abdominal distension are a problem.

Anyone who is taking aspirin or any other medication to thin the blood should avoid using *dong quai*.

Night sweats

These are the nocturnal version of a hot flush, and like the latter can vary greatly in frequency and severity. Some of us may find that we wake feeling no more hotter than usual and slightly damp, while those who are less fortunate may find that they wake at frequent intervals during the night feeling as though they are initially burning up, followed rapidly by a drenching sweat that leaves them feeling chilled and wringing wet.

If we are very unlucky and find that nights sweats fall into the second category, there are some simple steps we can take to improve the situation before we consider medication.

Quick-fix hints

- Make sure that bedrooms are well-ventilated and neither uncomfortably stuffy or too cold.
- Other factors that can contribute to a satisfying and sound night's sleep include sound-proofing bedrooms as much as possible, and blocking out light adequately by having effective curtains (but not so dark that they act as blackout curtains, since these can make getting up in the morning extra difficult).
- Avoid the foods and drinks listed in the 'Hot flushes' section, since anything that aggravates hot flushes can also make night sweats worse.
- Keep a bowl of tepid water, a sponge, a fresh towel and dry nightwear by the side of the bed. This means that we don't have the extra disturbance of getting out of bed to change if our nightwear has becoming wringing wet. By sponging down with tepid water after a severe night sweat we can also avoid the unpleasant feeling of stale perspiration lying on our skins.
- Make sure that bedding and nightwear are made from natural fibres such as cotton rather than synthetic blends including nylon.

- Cutting down drastically on red meat consumption may also be helpful in easing night sweats and hot flushes, since the hormones that are ingested with red meat can make hormone imbalances more severe. The same can also be true if consumption of dairy food is excessive.

Aromatherapy hints

Five or six drops of either of the following may be added to a warm bath or burnt in a vaporiser in order to ease night sweats: *clary sage* or *cypress*.

Homoeopathic hints

- Hot night sweats that alternate with severe chills which make us haul the bedclothes up and down all night may benefit greatly from a few doses of *pulsatilla*. Choice of this remedy would be confirmed by chilliness with a desire for fresh air and an extreme dislike of stuffy, badly ventilated surroundings.
- Night sweats that move in a wave-like motion through the body that are especially severe on waking may respond well to *lachesis*. Additional symptoms that would suggest that choice of this remedy is appropriate include an marked aversion (almost to the point of phobia) of anything tight worn around the neck. There also may be a real dislike of going to bed, with a tendency to stay up into the early hours of the morning, because of the unpleasant symptoms brought on by sleep.
- Very severe night sweats that lead to sleep deprivation with emotional and physical exhaustion during the day may do well in response to *sepia*. Selection of this remedy would be confirmed by irritability and depression as a result of feeling unable to cope with domestic and emotional demands. Night sweats move up the body with an unpleasant sense of dizziness and disorientation on waking.
- *Sulphur* may be an appropriate remedy to consider if night sweats are very severe. See profile of this remedy already given under the heading 'Hot flushes'.

Herbal hints

- *Black cohosh* may be as helpful in easing night sweats as hot flushes. See section on 'Hot flushes' for more information on this herb.
- *Hops* are claimed to have an oestrogen-balancing effect and as a result may be very beneficial where night sweats have appeared in response to a dramatic drop in oestrogen levels. *Hops* have been combined with *rhubarb root* in a product called Phytoestrol which is manufactured in Germany. It has been suggested that although it may not act as rapidly as conventional hormone replacement therapy, Phytoestrol appears to stimulate significant improvement in symptoms such as hot flushes and night sweats without severe side effects or toxic interaction with other drugs.
- *Chastetree* may also have a beneficial effect on hot flushes and night sweats as well as restoring a sense of emotional harmony and balance. Used daily, *chastetree* appears to enhance progesterone and dopamine production with the result that it can have a profoundly positive effect on mind, emotions and body. It can be taken in the form of capsules, infusions or tincture.

Anxiety and panic attacks

One of the surprising symptoms of menopause may be the abrupt emergence of feelings of unsettling anxiety, or even outright panic for which we may be completely unprepared. This is likely to be especially the case if we have seen ourselves as being calm and unruffled by nature, having the emotional reserves in the past to roll with whatever punches life may have thrown at us.

Some of us may have been aware during the years leading up to the menopause of a low-grade form of concern and anxiety. This may be connected to the experience of getting older with all of the physical and emotional changes that are involved in this inevitable process. For many of us, the challenges ahead may seem unwelcome and overwhelming, with the result that we may begin to feel a growing sense of anxiety that may become more acute from time to time in response to specific triggers (such as glancing in the mirror after a late night and seeing the face reflected back at us looking the worse for wear). Of course, more serious triggers can also emerge at this time, such as coming to terms with children maturing and being ready to start their own lives outside the family home, the death of parents (which can bring home to us the sense of our own mortality almost more than any other single event), or the breakup of a long-term relationship.

On the other hand, anxiety can also descend on those of us who feel life is going really well. After all, mid-life can be a time for many of us when we reap the rewards of hard-won experience at work and in personal relationships. Many of us may welcome the increased freedom these years can give us, when we truly have the sense of being our own person again as others are no longer as dependent on us as they were in the past. In these cases, the descent of anxiety as a menopausal symptom can feel especially alarming and troublesome, since there is no obvious cause for these unpleasant sensations.

Symptoms of anxiety can vary from one person to another, but the following are common features of the problem:

- Increased pulse rate
- Hyperventilation (breathing in a more rapid and shallow way from the upper chest)
- Nausea or actual vomiting in extreme cases
- Sweating
- Diarrhoea
- Dizziness and/or disorientation
- Waking from sleep with a start
- Tightness in the chest
- Muscle trembling
- Dry mouth
- Impaired memory and concentration

However unpleasant these symptoms are, it is very helpful to know that there are simple steps we can take to restore our emotional equilibrium and feel back in control in double-quick time. These may include the general positive lifestyle changes listed below to start with. If these alone don't improve the situation considerably it is well worth experimenting with some alternative medical self-help. If, on the other hand, you feel you are dealing with well-established patterns of anxiety that have developed steadily over many years, you are much more likely to benefit greatly from professional alternative medical treatment.

Quick-fix hints

Diaphragmatic breathing

When anxious feelings descend, take control by changing your breathing pattern. Many of us may not be aware that we instinctively begin to take short, shallow breaths when we feel anxious and tense. This pattern of breathing unfortunately makes us feel even worse, since the balance of oxygen and carbon dioxide in our bodies is adversely affected. The ironic result is that the more we breathe from our upper chest, the more uncomfortable and threatened we are likely to feel. The key to changing this situation and calming ourselves down quickly lies in learning how to breathe using our whole lung capacity. This invaluable tool to relaxation and clear-headedness is called diaphragmatic breathing and can be learned without great fuss, bother or paraphernalia.

Breathing for relaxation can be done most easily at first when lying on the floor or sitting in a straight-backed chair. Put your hand gently on your abdomen (just above the level of your navel) and take a couple of full breaths. As you breathe in, feel the air filling your lungs from the top to the bottom so that your hand should rise up and outwards as your lungs expand with air. When breathing out, your hand should sink down first as the lungs expel carbon dioxide from the base of the lungs to the tip. Take a few slow, steady breaths in this way and you should notice the hand resting on your belly gently rising and falling as you breathe fully in and out. Never force the breath, but try to make it as rhythmical and gentle as you can. If you feel light-headed or dizzy at any point, just take a few normal breaths and that should clear your head.

Once you know how it feels to do it properly, this is an invaluable technique that can be used at any time or anywhere when feelings of tension or anxiety descend. Of course, familiarity with how it feels to breathe from the abdomen means that you no longer need to lie down with your hand on your belly to do it well. As a result, you can use this relaxing breathing technique when you are sitting at a desk, driving, walking, or in bed. As a result, you have a powerful tool at your disposal that puts you in the driving seat once again, rather than feeling helpless and disempowered in the face of anxiety.

Meditation

If we have a history of established problems with anxiety or panic attacks, learning a simple meditation technique that can be practised each day can be extremely advantageous in helping us gain a generally calmer perspective on life. In order to meditate we need to sit in a straight-backed chair that supports our spine well in an upright position. If this feels distracting or uncomfortable in any way, try lying flat on the floor, or sitting on a cushion in a cross-legged position instead. Always make sure that whatever position you choose feels comfortable to you, since any physical discomfort may distract you from reaching a calm, meditative state. Your hands should feel loose and relaxed at your sides, your spine should be straight but not stiff and your head comfortably supported. Clothes should be warm (always bear in mind that body temperature can drop considerably while in an extremely relaxed and meditative state), and they should also be loose and unrestricting. Surroundings conducive to meditation should be peaceful, not too brightly or harshly lit, and well ventilated in order to avoid stuffiness which can lead to drowsiness (the latter is a different state to the form of deep relaxation that is entered as a result of meditation). Without initially changing anything, become slowly aware of your breathing rhythm and pattern. As time goes by, slowly and gently begin to regulate your breathing patterns, making them as steady and effortless as possible. It may help to visualise your breath as a wave that is ebbing and flowing to a gentle but steady rhythm, or as a balloon that is inflating and deflating with each inhalation and each exhalation. There may be other images that instinctively appeal to you: just choose whatever feels appropriate.

As you become in tune with your breathing pattern, repeat a sound or word slowly to yourself: try to clear your mind and focus exclusively on that sound. At first the chances are that distracting thoughts will spill into your mind, all competing for your attention. Don't get thrown or put off by this; just calmly put them to one side as they arise, and concentrate once again on your chosen sound or word. In time, this should get easier to do, but don't panic if it seems more difficult than you might have thought to clear your mind. Make meditation practice a regular part of your daily routine and you should find levels of concentration improve as you feel less inclined to feel anxious.

Avoiding certain foods and drinks

Certain foods and drinks have a reputation for aggravating symptoms of anxiety, and these are paradoxically the items that we may crave when feeling tense. They include foods containing a high proportion of refined sugar, chocolate, and drinks such as alcohol, strong tea, coffee and cola drinks that contain caffeine and a hefty amount of refined sugar. These items should ideally be removed from our diets or cut down dramatically, since they can be responsible for exaggerating sleep disturbance (which can also be a common menopausal symptom), while also elevating our risk of developing osteoporosis. Substitute fresh fruit and vegetable snacks where possible, as well as soya products, and small amounts of dairy foods (from an organic source where possible). Alternative drinks include herb teas or fruit-flavoured tisanes, fig-based coffee substitutes, decaffeinated coffee (ideally choose one that has removed the caffeine using a water-filtering process rather than a chemical solvent, since the latter may leave traces in the product), and herbal, fruit-flavoured, carbonated drinks that are not laden with added sugar. It is best to avoid carbonated drinks that are advertised as low calorie, 'healthy' products, since these can include a range of additives, colourings, artificial sweeteners and caffeine that can be positively unhealthy. They carry a particular threat to menopausal women because of their high phosphorus content which encourages calcium to leach from the bones, increasing our risk of osteoporosis.

Bedtime drinks

If recurrent anxiety is combined with insomnia, try taking a warm drink of hot milk, honey, and a pinch of cinnamon as a bedtime drink. On the other hand, this should be avoided if you suffer from asthma, sinus problems, or general congestion of the chest, since cow's milk can lead to increased mucus production.

Vitamin B complex

It can be helpful if anxiety is a long-standing problem to include foods in your diet that are high in B vitamins in order to provide maximum support for the nervous system. These include wheatgerm, green leafy vegetables, brewers' yeast, and blackstrap molasses.

Regular exercise

Consider taking up regular exercise as a way of easing anxiety by burning the excess adrenalin that is produced whenever we feel stressed or anxious. If adrenalin is produced in excess on a regular basis we enter a state of arousal that can contribute to symptoms of high blood pressure, poor sleep patterns or sleep quality, and digestive upsets such as indigestion, heartburn, diarrhoea and constipation. Regular, rhythmical physical exercise such as brisk walking, swimming, cycling, trampolining, dancing or running helps promote a calmer, clearer state of mind that can make us more confident of our physical and mental capabilities – something that is especially welcome when we approach and move through the menopause. Exercise that makes our hearts and lungs work more efficiently and at peak performance is especially beneficial as an all-round energy-booster and emotional balancer.

However, it's good to remember that regularity of sessions spent exercising is the most important thing if we are to reap maximum benefits from our chosen activity. In other words, it's less beneficial (and can be positively counter-productive) to exercise furiously for an hour every three weeks or so, rather than enjoying half an hour's activity five days a week. If we adopt the latter approach and keep it up, we are far more likely to see sustained physical and emotional improvements.

Aromatherapy hints

Have a regular aromatic, relaxing bath by adding five drops of any of the following to warm bath water: *bergamot, clary sage, lavender*, or *ylang ylang*. Any of these essential oils can also be burnt in a custom-made vaporiser in order to induce a calm, soothing atmosphere whenever nerves feel strained.

Homoeopathic hints

- A few doses of *aconite* can do a tremendous amount to calm feelings of extreme panic and terror that seem to descend out of the blue. Anxiety that responds decisively to *aconite* tends to involve panic attacks with an overwhelming fear of death. In an anxiety state, skin is either flushed and dry or it may alternate between sensations of heat and chill. It helps to know that *aconite* is a very fast-acting remedy that should yield a marked improvement with a few minutes of taking it. As a result, if it is the right remedy, no more than a couple of doses should be needed to calm symptoms down substantially.
- Anxiety that is connected to an overly stressful lifestyle with a tendency to rely on coffee, alcohol, cigarettes and painkillers to keep the pace may respond very positively to *nux vomica*. This remedy can be often indicated during the menopause, since this is often a time when women find that they can no longer tolerate alcohol, stimulants, and 'burning the candle at both ends' in the same way they did in the past. Additional symptoms that would confirm choice of this remedy would include irritability, regular hangover-type headaches, constipation, and poor sleep pattern.

- Panic attacks that come on at night with marked nausea and/or diarrhoea may be substantially relieved by taking a few doses of *arsenicum album*. Choice of this remedy would be confirmed by a marked tendency to feel anxious if established routines or feeling in control are threatened in any way. When anxious, any mess or untidiness in external surroundings can cause a disproportionate amount of distress.

Herbal hints

- *Lemon balm* has a reputation for calming the mind and promoting a state of overall mental, emotional and physical relaxation. It also appears to boost energy levels when the nervous system has been drained by excessive levels of stress. It can be taken as a herbal tea to induce a sound night's sleep, or in the morning when it acts as a refreshing drink to set us up for the demands of the day.
- *Oats* are well worth including in the diet on a regular basis because of the anxiety-reducing properties that they are thought to have. Easy ways of boosting oat intake include having a bowl of porridge each morning and choosing flapjacks instead of cakes when a sweet snack is needed.
- An infusion of any of the following may be used to ease symptoms of general tension and anxiety: *camomile, limeflower* and *valerian*. One teaspoon of dried herb should be added to a cup of hot water and left to brew in a covered container for approximately fifteen minutes. Once the liquid has cooled slightly, strain and sip as a soothing tea. However, always bear in mind that although *valerian* is a powerful, excellent remedy for easing the symptoms of tension, anxiety, insomnia and agitation, it is best avoided in large doses or over an extended period of time. Problems that can occur in association with either of these situations can include headaches, palpitations, or muscle spasms.
- If you prefer to take your herbs in tablet rather than tea form, you may prefer to take one of the proprietary brands of herbal tablets that can be used to relieve symptoms of anxiety or tension. They are likely to include *hops, valerian* and *gentian*. However,

they are to be avoided when pregnant or breast-feeding.

- Anxiety that is related to hot flushes may respond well to *motherwort*. This herb is thought to have a calming and balancing effect that can banish feelings of anxiety and relax tension, while also improving and harmonising energy levels. It can also be used as a preventive if you know that a particularly stressful or challenging event is at hand. For suggestions on how to take *motherwort*, see the 'Hot flushes' section.

Flower essences

Rescue remedy can be very effective in easing symptoms of anxiety and panic in double-quick time. A drop of two may be taken as required directly on the tongue, or four or five drops may be dissolved in a small glass of cold water and sipped when feelings of anxiety are present.

Sleep disturbance

One of the menopausal symptoms that can cause the most disruption and distress in women's lives is a tendency to disrupted sleep patterns and a reduction in sleep quality. This may be coped with more easily by those of us who have a well-established history of insomnia, while others who have always slept soundly may be appalled by the loss of refreshing, good quality sleep.

We cannot overestimate how essential a role sleep plays in ensuring that we achieve and maintain good quality health on mental, emotional and physical levels. When we sleep soundly for the optimum time to meet our individual requirements we give our vital organs a chance to rest, our immune systems have a much needed opportunity to recharge and renew themselves, while material from our subconscious can be explored safely through dreams. As a result, lack of sound, refreshing sleep can result in poor concentration, irritability, depression, fatigue, and a compromised ability to fight infection effectively.

If we suffer from night sweats as well as hot flushes during the menopause, extra problems can arise. It is clearly not going to help us have a restful sleep if we are woken at frequent intervals drenched in sweat. Sleep disturbance can take a variety of forms, but one of the most common patterns to emerge in connection to the menopause is to find that we fall asleep with little difficulty, but wake with infuriating regularity at 2 or 3 a.m. We may toss and turn for a couple of hours, only to find that we fall into a deep sleep around the time we should be waking up feeling refreshed and ready to face the day.

For those of us who have reservations about using sleeping tablets because of unwanted side effects of drowsiness during the day, possible dependence, and lack of effectiveness after prolonged use, it is tremendously important to realise that there are effective alternative measures that we can use in order to re-establish a sound night's sleep without relying on conventional sleeping tablets.

Quick-fix hints

- Make sure that you engage in some form of relaxing activity for a couple of hours before bedtime in order to allow your mind and body to switch off thoroughly. Above all else, it is best to avoid the temptation of doing a few hours of mental work before sleep: this only has the undesirable effect of making it harder for the brain to switch off when we need to rest.
- It often helps to have a regular routine that prepares mind and body for sleep. This needn't become fixed or rigid, but it can provide a loose framework within which the body and mind have a chance to relax and unwind. This could include a relaxation exercise, burning relaxing essential oils in a vaporiser, and/or reading.
- Avoid eating heavy meals late at night as a rule, and steer clear of strong tea, chocolate or coffee from late afternoon onwards if you know that you have a tendency to wake in the early hours of the morning. Alcohol should also be avoided in large quantities since it can have a stimulant effect which can prevent sleep, in addition to other health hazards that are known to be

related to a high alcohol consumption. Alternatively, a small glass of wine taken early in the evening with a light meal can have the opposite effect by helping us unwind and let go of the tensions of the day. This is partly due to the way that alcohol is released more slowly into the bloodstream when it is taken with food. However, if you have a history of pre-menstrual insomnia, it is best to avoid alcohol during this phase of your cycle, since this is a time when you are likely to be more vulnerable to the disruptive effects of alcohol on sleep pattern.

- Try to take some exercise in the fresh air each day (a walk at lunchtime can be enough to do the trick).
- Although many of us will be aware that we can eat specific foods to give us a much-needed energy boost at a low point in the day, it may come as a surprise that we can choose foods that have a sedative effect if we want to give ourselves the best chance of enjoying a sound night's sleep. These include avocado, peanut butter, dairy foods (because of their calcium content), lettuce, bananas (which include the antidepressant and relaxing action of tryptophan) and oranges (due to their bromine content which helps induce a relaxed state).
- If life has been especially stressful and demanding, learning how to meditate or getting to grips with an effective relaxation technique can do a great deal to help us calm down and achieve a good night's rest on a regular basis.
- See the 'Night sweats' section for additional advice that may help with sleep disturbance.

Aromatherapy hints

Massaging a soothing a blend of essential oils in a carrier oil into the skin may do a great deal to induce a relaxed state before bed. A suitable blend would include three drops of *camomile* and *mandarin* added to two teaspoons of carrier oil.

Homoeopathic hints

- If anxious insomnia is a problem, and there is a tendency to wake feeling tense and nervous around 2 a.m., a few doses of *arsenicum album* may be enough to re-establish a healthy sleep pattern. If this is the appropriate remedy, there will be a tendency to feel extremely restless and a compulsion to get out of bed and make a warm drink, in preference to tossing and turning in bed waiting for sleep to descend again.

- If exhaustion sets in to the point where one feels physically, mentally and emotionally drained with resulting lowered libido, *sepia* is worth consideration. This remedy can help break the vicious cycle of feeling exhausted and drowsy during the day, but infuriatingly wide awake at night. Headaches, queasiness and dizziness may become a recurrent feature due to permanent tiredness.

- If there is an aversion to going to bed because of the unpleasant feelings associated with falling asleep, or on waking, *lachesis* may do a great deal to ensure a relaxed night's rest. Choice of this remedy would be confirmed by a tendency to hold the breath when falling asleep, and waking with a sudden jolt or jerking sensation. Those who would benefit from *lachesis* feel psychologically and physically awful on waking.

- Those who have a tendency to rely on alcohol, painkillers or sedatives in order to fall asleep should consider *nux vomica* as a possibility. If this remedy is indicated there will be general features of having problems in switching off from stresses at work and/or domestic worries. *Nux vomica* can greatly benefit those who are high achievers, who push themselves too hard, and who have to rely on chemical 'props' such as caffeine, alcohol and/or cigarettes in order to keep the pace. Common physical symptoms that benefit from *nux vomica* include headaches, constipation, and indigestion.

- Sleeplessness with great physical discomfort at night including feeling constantly uncomfortably either overheated or chilled may benefit greatly from *pulsatilla*, provided other features agree. These would include a general tendency to be weepy from lack of sleep and in great need of sympathetic company. One feels very drowsy on going to bed, but wakes in the early hours of the morning just as a night sweat is about to start.

Herbal hints

- Use an infusion of the following herbs that can be added to a warm bath in order to relax body and mind as a preparation for sleep. Take three generous handfuls of any of the following and add them to a small pan of cold water, leave to stand overnight, bring to the boil, and strain: *lavender, limeflower, camomile,* or *passionflower.*

- The beneficial effects of relaxing and sleep-inducing herbs may also be enjoyed in herbal tea form. Always choose flavours that appeal to your palate rather than regarding what you are drinking as medicine, since the experience needs to be pleasurable as well as relaxing! Possible herbs include *camomile, limeflower,* or *passionflower.* You can use commercially prepared tea bags or, when using fresh herbs, add one teaspoon to a cup of hot water. Cover the liquid and leave to stand for fifteen minutes before straining and sipping as a soothing bedtime drink.

- Poor sleep pattern that results in a general state of nervous restlessness may be greatly improved by taking *avena sativa compound* on a regular basis until symptoms improve. The tincture contains *valerian, passionflower, hops, oats,* and a homoeopathic dilution of *coffee.* Twenty drops may be diluted in a small glass of cold water and taken before bed.

Fatigue

Feeling we could do with more energy can be a concern at any stage of life, but the years leading up to and following the menopause can be a particular time when we may feel at a low physical ebb. This is partly due to the physical changes that are going on at a hormonal level, with oestrogen and progesterone levels dropping steadily. It can also be linked to a range of other factors that are likely to emerge at this time. These may include changes in pace of life and demands being made on us professionally and personally, psychological challenges linked to the whole issue of getting older, changes in sleep pattern and quality (see 'Night sweats' and 'Sleep disturbance' sections for more information), and adapting to new dietary needs and considerations in order to give our minds and bodies maximum support and resilience.

On the other hand, it halps enormously to realise that there are positive steps we can take to make the years of this vital transition as smooth as possible. Once we begin to work with the changing rhythms of our bodies we have the best chance of living life to its full energetic potential. In fact, we may be surprised to find that once we experience our optimum 'cruising level' of energy, we have more resources of vitality at our disposal than we might have thought possible.

It helps at the outset to establish that when we talk about energy within a holistic context, we are considering the full spectrum of the energy experience including mental, emotional and physical well-being. In other words, when we are enjoying our maximum experience of vitality we should find that not only do we have more sustained levels of physical energy at hand on a day-to-day level, but we should also discover that our emotions flow more smoothly with fewer ups and downs, as well as enjoying improved levels of concentration.

This may all sound like a tall order, especially if we are dreading the onset of the menopause because we fear that we may be falling apart. However, once we begin to understand that a great deal of this fear is rooted in feeling powerless in the face of an inevitable series of changes, appreciating that there are vital steps we can take to support ourselves through these transformations can be immensely empowering and confidence-boosting. As a result, what was the source of unmanageable fear and anxiety can become a challenge that can spur us on to care for ourselves in a way that we may not have previously considered relevant or realistic.

Quick-fix hints

Sound sleep

The cornerstone of sustained, high-quality energy is a sound night's sleep. There is no magic number of hours that we should sleep each night, since what suits one of us may be totally unsuitable for another. In other words, some of us may instinctively be aware that if we don't have a solid eight hours rest we feel less than human, while this may feel soporific and counter-productive to someone who thrives on a maximum of six solid hours each night. If we have experienced a marked negative change in our sleep patterns as a consequence of the menopause, this can have a noticeable knock-on effect in making us feel drained and unrefreshed during the day. If this has happened in response to a lack of ability to switch off when bedtime comes, or the additional rest-wrecker of night sweats, we can take steps to improve the situation. These are to be found in the 'Sleep disturbance' and 'Night sweats' sections (pp. 152–6 and 142–4).

The food that we eat

The quality of energy that we experience can be directly influenced by the nature of the food that we eat on a regular basis. One of the most noticeable factors in influencing our levels of mental, emotional and physical energy is whether we have a tendency to go for the 'quick-fix' solution when feeling low. 'Quick-fix' foods and drinks include strong tea, coffee, sugary snacks like chocolate bars, cakes or biscuits, crisps, fizzy drinks and 'junk foods' in general that are usually highly processed and bear little resemblance to any food in its fresh, natural, unprocessed state.

Unfortunately, although these foods and drinks are very convenient to eat as snacks on the run, they have the disadvantage of playing havoc with our blood sugar levels. Most of them will initially give a sugar-induced rush of energy, which is rapidly followed by a sense of fatigue and exhaustion when blood sugar levels plummet as the pancreas secretes insulin. There is also the additional problem that the foods and drinks listed above can lead to our feeling tense, jittery and anxious in addition to feeling washed out. They can also have the disadvantage of aggravating sleep problems and making hot flushes more severe.

On the other hand, foods that give us a sustained, high-quality experience of energy right across the board are also foods that we need at menopause in order to minimise common problems such as hot flushes, night sweats and mood swings. These include wholegrain foods such as brown rice and wholemeal bread, pasta, pulses, small amounts of dairy foods, organic poultry, fish, vegetables, fruit and soya products. By enjoying foods that are as close to their natural state as possible (in other words where additives and preservatives have not been used) we are able to avoid the ingredients that can aggravate menopausal symptoms. Smoked or preserved foods such as salami and smoked meats are known to have a high proportion of phosphorus as well as being high in saturated fat. The latter can increase our risk of heart disease when taken in excess, while the former can aggravate a tendency to osteoporosis by adversely affecting uptake of calcium. By choosing complex carbohydrates such as wholegrains and potatoes we are most likely to experience a steady, slow release of energy because complex carbohydrates take longer to digest than their refined counterparts.

A swifter energy release may be occasionally gained by eating a couple of pieces of fruit. Although fruit sugar (fructose) is more readily broken down than complex carbohydrates, it is still less likely to cause as much instability in blood sugar levels as table sugar (sucrose). The end result is that we can afford to use fruit as an energy-boosting snack if we feel we are flagging, since it's less likely than a chocolate bar to set off a sugar rush followed quickly by exhaustion. Looking at practicalities as well, it's clearly much easier to eat an apple or a banana in a five-minute break than a plate of brown rice and beans.

Don't be put off by thinking that moving into eating for sustained energy and stamina is just too radical, because it must be done at one stroke. This is just not true, and might even be counter-productive since it could result in an unwelcome shock to the system. In order to obtain the most lasting and sustainable positive results it is best to slowly substitute complex carbohydrates for the refined products that are already on your shelves. In this way, stocks of wholemeal flour and pasta can replace refined varieties as these are used up, and sugar-free muesli can be bought as stocks of refined breakfast cereal go down.

Caffeinated drinks

In any discussion of energy production, it helps enormously if we begin to understand how coffee and other caffeinated drinks affect our systems. Many of us will have got firmly into the habit of reaching for a strong cup of coffee when we fell that we are mentally and physically tired and need a quick energy 'fix'. It is certainly true that a hefty dose of caffeine will give us an initial boost and temporarily make us feel clear-headed but, sadly, this is only the start of the story.

Coffee has a major destabilising effect on our blood sugar levels (this is made even worse when we take our coffee with a hefty helping of sugar, chocolate bar or a sticky cake), which gives us a temporary 'lift' only to leave us crashing down an hour or two later, craving for more. Although we may feel that a cup of strong coffee is the answer when we need a mental 'edge' to help us deal with a pressing demand or deadline, this impression is only partly true. In reality, although we may feel mentally sharper after a coffee, the truth is that tests have demonstrated that coffee can create confusion and jitteriness in high dosage that can interfere with clarity of thought and decision-making abilities. Additional problems with regular coffee-drinking include recurrent head-aches, disturbed sleep, raised blood pressure, increased risk of osteoporosis, anxiety and dependence. See the 'Quick-fix' section in 'Anxiety and panic attacks' (pp. 146–50) for general advice on alternative drinks.

Eating patterns

Eating patterns can also affect our energy patterns by determining whether we have peaks and troughs or a steady flow of energy. One of the simplest ways of ensuring that we avoid low blood sugar levels (which can make us feel tired, light-headed and lacking in concentration) is to avoid going for long periods of time without eating. Try to eat something light and digestible every couple of hours: a few pieces of fruit, salad vegetables, or a seasoned brown rice cake with a savoury topping would be ideal. It also helps if we avoid the temptation to skip a meal in the hope that we will get more work done in the time that we would have spent eating. If we do this on a regular basis, there is a strong chance that we will eventually become 'burnt out' mentally, emotionally and physically owing to lack of a relaxing space within which to unwind.

Time to relax

In order to enjoy maximum levels of energy and vitality we need to allow ourselves enough space and time within which we can relax and recharge our energy batteries. This is not a luxury but a necessity if we want to experience our optimum level of vitality and alertness on a daily basis. Relaxation techniques can be a vital tool in empowering us to reflect and let go within the context of a busy, pressured life. Take advantage of the increasing number of audio cassette tapes that are appearing on the market which will talk you through a guided relaxation. Once the basic skill has been mastered it is worth making sure that a little time is set aside each day for conscious relaxation. By doing this on a daily basis, the chances are that you will develop a keen sense of awareness of the areas of your body where you are holding tension. This can be discovery of vital importance, since we can waste energy that could be put to positive use when we keep muscles permanently clenched and in a low-level state of discomfort.

Breathing

Breathing is also one of the basic tools we can use in order to give ourselves an immediate energy boost by enabling us to make maximum use of the oxygen that we breathe in. Make sure that you breathe out fully as you exhale, so that maximum use is made of your lung capacity. It is worth making a special effort to become aware of breathing techniques if you feel tense or anxious as well as tired, since feeling stressed can result in our breathing pattern becoming undesirably rapid and shallow. This has the adverse 'knock-on' effect of causing an imbalance of carbon dioxide and oxygen in our bodies. By adapting our breathing pattern to make it slower, deeper and more even, we can give ourselves the maximum chance of feeling clear-headed, calmer and more in control. If you are interested in developing more awareness of breathing techniques for increased energy and/or relaxation, consider attending a yoga class.

Dry skin brushing

Chronic lethargy and sluggish energy levels may be improved by regular skin-brushing techniques. Dry skin brushing can be an effective way of stimulating our lymphatic systems and encouraging efficient elimination of toxic waste from the skin. By encouraging smooth functioning of our lymphatic systems we can help our bodies detoxify, which can have the dual effect of improving energy levels as well as protecting ourselves from recurrent infections. Dry skin brushing is simple and straightforward to learn: all that is needed is a dry hemp mitt or a natural bristle brush (avoid nylon or other synthetic bristles which will not do the job efficiently). Use firm, but not harsh sweeping strokes, moving in an upward direction towards the trunk on the arms and legs, and down the torso. Avoid brushing any areas of skin that are broken, inflamed or sensitive, and take a bath or shower following a skin-brushing session in order to remove toxic debris from the surface of the skin.

Aromatherapy hints

Essential oils that have a stimulating, invigorating effect include *rosemary, peppermint, coriander* and *grapefruit*. Five or six drops may be added to a warm bath or vaporised in a custom-made essential-oil burner for an instant energy boost.

Homoeopathic hints

- Lowered energy levels and general muscular aching that follow overdoing physical activity in a frantic, 'last-ditch' effort to get fit may be greatly eased and relieved by a few doses of *arnica*. Symptoms that would confirm this choice include generalised muscular aching from head to foot (even passing water may feel painful as internal muscles also feel sore and strained), a feeling of extreme restlessness at night and inability to find a comfortable position in bed, and an overwhelming sense of exhaustion.

- Physical and mental exhaustion that follow a period of 'burning the candle at both ends' often respond swiftly and well to a few doses of *nux vomica*. This remedy can be enormously helpful when we discover to our dismay that we can no longer tolerate alcohol in the way that we used to, or even that having a night out seems to take a disproportionate toll on our sense of well-being and overall vitality. Additional symptoms that respond well to *nux vomica* include extreme irritability, a hangover-type headache, an overall feeling of queasiness, constipation, and a general sense of toxic overload.

- A sense of fatigue with extreme restlessness that presents relaxation and recuperation may call for *arsenicum album*. When this remedy is needed, there is likely to be a tendency for anxiety to set in as soon as any sense of being in control is challenged. Those who respond well to this remedy often take refuge in constantly trying to control their surroundings by always organising themselves and others. Tidiness and cleanliness may become obsessive, with a genuine feeling of distress setting in when circumstances prevent tidying up being done.

- Extreme fatigue that is combined with feeling emotionally flat and marked loss of libido may be relieved by *sepia*. When this remedy is strongly indicated, profound physical, emotional and mental tiredness is combined with a sense of apathy and indifference to everything and everyone, especially close family members who are perceived as making unreasonable demands. When *sepia* is needed there may be an initial aversion to making any physical effort, but once under way, rhythmic, vigorous exercise is the one thing that can create a sense of temporary invigoration.

- If easy exhaustion has been a long-term feature, combined with a generally sluggish metabolism and a tendency to easy weight gain after the menopause, taking *calc carb* may do a great deal to improve the situation. Additional problems that respond very well to this remedy include chilliness, chronic constipation, easy perspiration on making the slightest physical effort or feeling embarrassed, and inefficient circulation leading to severe chilliness alternating with uncomfortable flushes of heat. Unlike *sepia*, the symptoms that can be treated by *calc carb* tend to get worse as a result of physical exercise of any kind.

Herbal hints

- An infusion of any of the following dried herbs may be added to a warm bath in order to revive and invigorate mind and body: *rosemary* or *peppermint*. In order to make the infusion add three generous handfuls of herb to a pan of cold water. Leave to infuse overnight before bringing to the boil the next day. Strain, and add to a warm bath whenever a vitality boost is needed.
- The following herbs have a reputation for acting as effective nervous restoratives which may restore flagging energy levels when a state of 'burn-out' seems immanent: *wild oats, ginseng, skullcap* or *vervain*. They can be obtained and taken in tincture, tablet, or infusion form.
- If energy levels are flagging due to an inability to relax and unwind, with additional problems with sleep disturbance, it is worth considering *passionflower* or *valerian* as herbal preparations that can induce a calmer, more relaxed state and improve sleep patterns. However, it's best not to continue taking *varlerian* indefinitely, but to take it in short courses in order to avoid possible side effects such as headaches.

Flower essences

Extreme fatigue that sets in as a result of taking on too many professional responsibilities while also dealing with challenging demands at home may benefit from *elm*. When this flower essence is appropriate there may be as strong sensation of being mentally and physically unable to cope because of the sheer volume of work that has piled up. In order to make up a treatment bottle, fill a sterilised 1oz (28g) dropper bottle with still mineral water to which two drops of your selected flower essence may be added. Once a teaspoonful of brandy has been added, you have your stock bottle made up and ready for use. Take four drops diluted in a small glass of cold water four times a day. Hold the liquid in your mouth for a few seconds in order to give the remedy the maximum chance of being effective.

Fluid retention

Many of us may have experienced problems with periodic fluid retention if we have an established history of pre-menstrual syndrome (PMS). When PMS-related fluid retention is severe, tightness and swelling may be felt in the feet, ankles, tops of the thighs, waist, belly and fingers. The swelling may often build slowly in intensity until a period begins, when it begins to disperse. As the excess fluid drains from the tissues we are likely to find that we have a drastically increased urine output for a short while. There are other possible situations that may give rise to problems with fluid retention. These may include long-term tendencies to varicose veins, kidney problems, coronary heart disease, or taking medication that includes fluid retention as one of its side effects. If any of these factors are present, always seek a medical opinion rather than attempting self-help treatment that could easily lead us out of our depth.

As we reach menopause, we may find that fluid retention, instead of ceasing as a problem, can become a more established feature. If this is the case, there are a number of simple steps that we can take on a day-to-day basis in order to improve the situation. In addition, if extra help is needed in the short term in order to deal with a particularly noticeable episode of fluid retention, there are effective acute alternative medical measures that are listed below. However, it is important to bear in mind that these really are short-term strategies and, as a result, should not be depended upon to resolve a more established, recurrent, or severe problem. If the latter is the case, it is much more appropriate to seek help from a trained alternative practitioner who will attempt to address your predisposition to the problem with a view to eradicating rather than suppressing it.

Quick-fix hints

- If you have a general tendency to slight fluid retention from time to time it may help to include plenty of potassium-rich foods in your diet which act as a gentle diuretic. Suitable foods include vegetables, salads, raw fruit and freshly squeezed juices.
- Make a point of avoiding foods and drinks that have a reputation for aggravating fluid retention. These include: coffee, tea, alcohol, dairy foods, and 'instant' or convenience foods.
- Always avoid the temptation to snack on salty foods such as crisps or salted nuts, since table salt (sodium) stimulates the body to retain water in the tissues. Also beware of convenience foods that are likely to contain a large amount of sodium as well as a range of additional chemical additives and preservatives that can undermine our overall health. When seasoning foods, opt for ground, roasted sesame or sunflower seeds, or herbs that have a strong flavour such as rosemary or basil (these may be used fresh or dried and ground up) instead of using table salt.
- In any discussion of management of fluid retention, it helps to bear in mind that our bodies are made up of approximately 80 per cent water. Although it may sound obvious, we need to make a point of drinking enough water each day to support the fluid-eliminating function of our kidneys. Unfortunately, some of us may respond to signs of fluid retention by thinking that we should drink less water in order to reduce the problem.

This course of action has the undesirable effect of making the problem worse, since our bodies respond to the reduced intake of fluid by hanging on to reserves, making fluid retention more severe. On the other hand, drinking more water has the desirable effect of flushing excess fluid from our tissues and supporting the eliminating function of our kidneys. Try where possible to drink filtered or still mineral water, avoiding tap water unless there is no alternative.

- If a generally sluggish circulation is adding to problems with fluid retention, it may help to raise the legs while resting. In addition, regular, rhythmical exercise (such as walking) taken on a daily basis can encourage efficient working of the pump action of the calf muscles.

Homoeopathic hints

- Periodical bouts of fluid retention where the breasts feels taut and puffy may improve greatly after a dose or two of *apis*. Tissues around the eyes may look pale, rosy-red, puffy and water-logged. Areas of fluid retention that respond well to this remedy will 'pit' (leave a pale indentation that takes a while to spring back into shape) when gentle pressure is applied. Marked symptoms that suggest that the choice of this remedy is appropriate include lack of thirst and a severe sensitivity to warmth in any form. However, contact with cool compresses or cool air makes the affected area feel more comfortable, and waterlogged tissues are drained by movement.

- If fluid retention is a problem, with a history of craving for salt and savoury foods in general, then *nat mur* may be the appropriate remedy. Additional features that confirm this choice of remedy include dryness of the vagina, recurrent problems with cold sores, and a tendency to dry, sensitive skin. Symptoms are more severe after a period, or when overheated, and are greatly relieved by cool bathing, massage and sweating.

- Swelling that mostly affects the feet, on the other hand, may respond better to *arsenicum album*. Puffiness and fluid retention in the feet are likely to be combined with a sensation of 'restless legs' that may be especially troublesome at night. Feet feel numb and weary when swollen, and are worse from cold conditions and drinking alcohol. Warmth, gentle movement, and sweating all ease symptoms.

Herbal hints

Several herbs are thought to have natural diuretic qualities. These include *parsley, dandelion, oats* and *elderflower*. These may be incorporated quite easily in your diet on a day-to-day basis by using fresh *parsley* liberally as a seasoning, having a helping of porridge each day, and using *elderflower* as a soothing drink that helps us relax as well as enhancing the eliminatory and detoxifying action of the kidneys.

Loss of libido

Loss of libido is by no means inevitable after the menopause – in fact, many of us may find that we feel liberated by the freedom from the concerns of finding and maintaining the most appropriate, effective and safe form of contraception. As anxieties over accidental pregnancies fade into the background, love-making can become more spontaneous than ever before. This is combined with the way that many of us, around the time of the menopause, will have children who have become mature and left home, with the result that there is also likely to be more privacy than in previous years.

What happens to our sex drive leading up to, and following menopause will often have more to do with the quality of our intimate relationships and our levels of self-esteem and sense of 'fitting our skins' than merely being limited to a question of fluctuating hormone levels. In other words, there are undoubtedly physical symptoms that can occur at menopause that may affect our levels of sexual desire, such as dryness of the vagina and easily occurring urinary infections. But there are also deeper issues to be considered, such as the ease with which we can communicate with our sexual partners. If this has been a problem area for much of the time spent in the relationship, it is likely to be thrown into much sharper focus as we get older.

Generally speaking, libido is also closely related to the amount of energy that we have at our disposal. Whenever we feel unwell, we are likely to notice that we are less likely to take enjoyment in those things that normally give us sensual pleasure. We are less sensitive to and attracted by tastes, smells and sensations than we are when enjoying optimum health. As a result, is it any surprise that our libido may also feel less than flourishing at times like these? If feeling under par goes on for long enough, this can have a general undermining effect on our sex drive, which in turn often leads to a general concern and stress over the fact that we no longer feel as responsive as we think we should do.

Thankfully, there are general steps listed below that we can take in order to boost a temporarily flagging libido. If these do not promote a significant or lasting improvement, or if there is a short-lived improvement that keeps relapsing and running out of steam, it is well worth seeking help from an alternative medical practitioner. As always, they will be attempting to provide a whole body, mind and emotional treatment that boosts your whole system back on its course to maximum health and vitality.

Quick-fix hints

A general aversion to, or lack of interest in making love may develop as a result of growing physical discomfort during inter-course in the years approaching or following the menopause. This commonly becomes a problem if the walls of the vagina become thinned, dry, and more prone to inflammation and uncomfortable sensitivity as result. However, although this sounds rather depressing, it is important to realise that there are a range of practical self-help alternative measures that can be used to relieve the situation to a great extent. These include:

- Avoiding cosmetic preparations and toiletries that have a reputation for aggravating vaginal irritation and soreness.

Possible popular culprits include vaginal sprays, deodorants, talcs, highly perfumed soaps, deodorised sanitary protection, and strongly coloured or perfumed foam baths.

- Never apply soapy lather inside the vagina since it is totally unnecessary, and it also can contribute to further dryness, irritation and inflammation of the delicate tissues of the vagina.
- Vitamin E oil can be applied to sensitive vaginal areas in order to promote elasticity of the tissues and to soothe soreness.
- Never rush sexual foreplay, since the longer the time spent on becoming aroused, the better the chance we have of the vagina becoming well lubricated with resulting reduced likelihood of pain and discomfort.
- If dryness has become a well-established problem, apply a generous amount of lubricating gel to the interior and entrance of the vagina before making love.

Diet

If libido is flagging, consider the overall quality of your diet, making sure it is a rich enough supply of the essential nutrients that are needed for preserving a healthy sex drive. These include the following items: seafood, oysters, herrings, wholegrains, nuts, seeds, ginger, peppers, cloves, rosemary, parsley and garlic. Don't forget that the B complex vitamins also play an important role within this context. Foods rich in this vitamin group include dairy foods, wholegrains, pulses, beans, nuts, dark leafy vegetables and offal.

Stress

Try to realistically evaluate how much stress you have to deal with on a daily basis, since a healthy sex drive is often one of the first things to suffer when we feel that we are struggling to cope with demands that are made on us on a day-to-day basis. For techniques on how best to deal with stress-related problems see the section on 'Anxiety and panic attacks' (pp. 144–52).

Unresolved problems

If you feel that problems with lowered libido are linked to long-standing, unresolved problems between yourself and your sexual partner, counselling may be very helpful in enabling you to explore, develop positive insights and eventually come to terms with whatever issues lie at the root of your conflict. Organisations such as Relate that work with couples in order to identify areas of discord in their relationship can provide the framework that is needed to work through problems in a non-judgmental, supportive, insightful, neutral environment.

Depression

Diminished libido can be a common symptom of depression. If you have a past history of depression, or if you are experiencing a number of the following symptoms it would be worth discussing your problems with your GP or alternative health practitioner. Common symptoms of depression include:

- Poor sleep pattern with anxiety or feelings of depression on waking.
- Loss of appetite or comfort eating.
- Early waking.
- Low physical, mental and emotional energy causing problems with concentration and memory.

Aromatherapy hints

Sensual oils may be diffused in a custom-made vaporiser to stimulate an ailing libido. Alternatively, any of the following may be added to a warm bath or added to a carrier oil and used to give or receive a sensual massage: *clary sage, rose, geranium*, or *ylang ylang*. When using essential oils for a fragrant bath, add five to six drops of oil after running the bath and disperse the perfumed oil gently in the warm water. A medium concentration massage oil may be made by adding two or three drops of essential oil to every 5 ml of carrier oil.

Homoeopathic hints

- If lack of libido is associated with a growing sense of lack of confidence and lowered levels of self-esteem, *lycopodium* is worth considering. Choice of this remedy would be suggested by a tendency to cover up insecurities by adopting a harsh, critical and domineering approach to others as a way of diverting attention away from feeling vulnerable. Lowered libido may be made more of a problem by a persistent burning discomfort in the vagina that makes any attempt at intercourse less pleasurable than it should be.

- Total lack of interest in sex that is the result of feeling completely wiped out and mentally, emotionally and physically exhausted is likely to respond well to *sepia*. When this remedy is needed, there is a tendency to alternate between feeling low, lacking in motivation and energy, and extreme irritability. Domestic responsibilities and demands feel intolerable owing to lack of energy, and there is a general tendency to feel unable to cope. Along with mental and emotional hypersensitivity there is often a corresponding soreness, itching and uncomfortable sensitivity of the vaginal area.

- Lowered libido that follows invasive procedures such as laparoscopy, cone biopsy or hysterectomy may improve greatly by taking *staphisagria*. Reactions to surgery may involve feeling violated, especially if not enough information was given before the procedure was carried out. Sharp, stinging pains of the genital area may be a nagging problem, while love-making may be inevitably followed by a bout of cystitis. Suppressed anger may also benefit greatly from accurate prescription of this remedy.

Herbal hints

- *Peppermint* tea has been claimed to have aphrodisiac properties. The fresh herb may be used in an infusion, or ready-prepared teabags may be obtained that are made from the dried plant.
- *Ginger* is also considered to be a general tonic that can improve flagging sex drive that is due to a general state of exhaustion. The fresh spice can be used as a seasoning and infused in hot water to make a warming drink.
- If lowered libido is linked to having to deal with an excess of

stress, *wild oats*, *vervain* and *lemon balm* are effective herbs in supporting the nervous system.

- A general aversion to lovemaking that is related to pain and sensitivity linked to thinning of the walls of the vagina may respond well to *dong quai*. For more information on this herb see the 'Hot flushes' section on pp. 141–42.

Mood swings and depression

Erratic mood swings and generally feeling emotionally low can happen to us at any phase of our lives such as puberty, during and following pregnancy, or leading up to and following the menopause. What all of these life events have in common is that they each involve significant surges in hormone levels that can have a profound effect on our emotional and mental balance, as well as being responsible for noticeable and obvious physical changes.

There are additional factors apart from dwindling oestrogen levels that may be associated with the years approaching and following the menopause. These can also contribute to feelings of sadness, anxiety and general emotional instability. Some of these issues are covered in the 'Anxiety and panic attacks' section on pp. 144–52. Pressures that often arise at this time are linked to coming to terms with children maturing, becoming independent and leaving home. If we have put most of our energies into bringing up and meeting the needs of our families, this can leave us feeling despondent, lost and bereft as our children no longer need the care and attention we have been used to providing when they were younger.

Those of us who have chosen to put a career before family life may also experience an unwelcome emotional uneasiness by the time we are well into our forties if we have constantly put off the decision to have children. By this stage we are likely to have to come to terms with the fact that our bodies will have made the final decision for us, since fertility levels drop dramatically by the time we are into our forties.

As we make the transition from our forties to our fifties, this can be an emotionally difficult time, since ageing parents are also often needing more care and attention from us. If we are feeling physically and emotionally strong and resilient this can be an especially rewarding role to play, but if we are feeling psychologically needy ourselves it can feel an uneasy burden to have to carry.

Clearly, the years approaching and following the menopause form a watershed during which we need to find effective ways to support and nurture ourselves, so that we make it to the other side of this transitional phase stronger and wiser than we were before. However challenging this time of life may be, always remember that we have a host of practical alternative measures at our disposal that can support us in making this vitally important transition as smoothly as possible. However, if you have a history of previous depressive illness (perhaps following a pregnancy or series of stressful life events) it is extremely important to seek professional medical help from your alternative health practitioner and/or GP in order to ensure that you have the maximum amount of professional support at your disposal. For a quick run down of symptoms that suggest you may be suffering from depression see the check list in the section on 'Loss of libido' (p. 171).

Quick-fix hints

Expressing feelings

If you feel you need to gain a better perspective on your emotional situation, it can be extremely helpful to express your feelings in the company of someone with whom you feel extremely at ease and relaxed. This could be anyone from a close friend, family member, or family doctor. Alternatively, you may feel less inhibited and more at ease speaking frankly about difficult feelings and emotions with someone you have never met before such as a counsellor. However, it is important not to overlook the importance of also speaking honestly with your partner about how you are feeling, since it is sometimes easy to overlook the other person who is also most closely involved in your personal situation.

If you feel able to explore feelings of anger, vulnerability, insecurity, or confusion about your family moving on, you are giving your partner a vital opportunity to be equally honest about their emotional reaction to the same situation. This can be especially valuable if they are approaching retirement, since this is a frequently traumatic time when feelings of insecurity or anxiety about the future can descend. By exploring avenues of communication at this watershed in both of your lives, you may also be opening up avenues of renewed closeness and intimacy as you experience a shared understanding of your changing situation.

Exploring fresh challenges

As your domestic situation moves on, try focusing on exploring fresh challenges or developing interests that may have been laid to one side due to shortage of time in the past. By becoming involved in new physical or mental occupations such as taking an adult education course, becoming physically fit by joining a gym, taking up a yoga course, or doing voluntary work, you may be surprised to find yourself exploring fresh horizons at a time when you least expected it. As a result of this process, you may find yourself regarding the middle phase of your life as part of an upward spiral rather than the beginning of a negative downward trend. Taking this proactive approach to new interests also enables us to make new friends who may be in a similar situation to us. This can also provide us with a positive antidote to unwelcome feelings of loneliness and isolation that are common reactions to facing the challenge of changing family dynamics.

Trying new ways of cooking

Make a concerted effort to explore fresh new ways of cooking if you feel that you have been relying too much on convenience foods and 'quick-fix' snacks instead of proper meals. The years leading up to and following the menopause are a phase of life when we need more support than ever from a nutritious diet if we are to function at our best on mental, emotional and physical levels. Junk the convenience foods wherever possible, and focus on making imaginative and plentiful helpings of fresh vegetables and salads an essential focus of main meals. Maximum vitamin content can be preserved by steaming or stir-frying: these methods of cooking have the added advantage of keeping the fresh, crisp texture of vegetables. Avoid regular portions of red meat, smoked items, coffee, alcohol, salty snacks, dehydrated 'instant' soups, full-fat dairy products, and foods or fizzy drinks that include hefty helpings of sugar. Not only do these foods often contribute to unpleasant mood swings, but they can also aggravate a tendency to develop two of the most common causes of anxiety in the years following the menopause: osteoporosis and heart disease. Experiment instead with home-made Indian dishes that combine pulses with rice (making sure that you go easy on the spices if hot flushes are a problem), Chinese dishes that highlight stir-fried vegetables with small helpings of seafood, chicken or fish.

Checking on regular consumption of addictive substances

If mood swings are becoming an obvious or worrying part of your day-to-day experience, it can be revealing to realistically evaluate the amount of addictive, or mood-altering substances that you take on a daily basis. Quite apart from the obvious 'bad guys', such as recreational or hard drugs like heroin, consider the 'soft' or more socially acceptable addictive substances. These include chocolate, sugar, caffeine (not only in tea or coffee but also fizzy drinks and 'natural' sources such as gurana), painkillers containing a combination of paracetamol and codeine, cigarettes and alcohol.

If most or all of these are taken on a daily basis, there is a strong chance that they are going to contribute to marked or severe mood swings. However, if you are shocked to find out how many of these you take on a regular basis, don't panic and be tempted to go on a radical 'cold turkey' regime, since this is likely to make you feel pretty unwell while your system tries to cope without the stimulating or relaxing effect of a combination of these items. You are more likely to reach a successful conclusion if you concentrate on the item that you are obviously dependent upon, and steadily eliminate this item initially from your daily diet. For example, if coffee is your main addiction (this can be established easily by asking yourself how you would feel if you were deprived of it), it's best not to cut it out overnight, or unpleasant symptoms of caffeine withdrawal are likely to follow. Try instead to replace a few cups of coffee with a decaffeinated version and/or coffee substitute. Herbal or fruit teas can also be used in order to give more variety. Steadily phase out caffeinated coffee in this way and you should find that you are less likely to experience symptoms of withdrawal.

On the other hand, if coffee holds little attraction, but you find you really have more of an attachment to alcohol, and especially if you feel that your intake has been steadily building recently, be honest about how much you are having on a daily basis. If this is not easily within the recommended weekly allowance (fourteen units for women), you may need professional help in order to deal effectively with the situation. Alternatively, if your alcohol intake has been sneaking up recently in response to a stressful situation, but nevertheless still remains within your weekly allowance, mood swings will benefit greatly from cutting down on your consumption of alcohol overall. Make a start by substituting for a glass of wine or measure of spirits a non-sugary, herbal-flavoured soft drink, unsweetened fruit juice, or mineral water with a twist of lemon or lime. Again, there's no reason to feel you absolutely have to go 'cold turkey' and become teetotal overnight, but by steadily increasing the amount of non-alcoholic drinks that you consume it is easy to halve the amount of alcohol that is being drunk with very little effort needing to be made. Even if your alcohol intake is on the modest side it's a very good idea to have a couple of alcohol-free nights each week in order to give your liver a much-needed opportunity to rest and regenerate itself.

Once these guidelines are in place you may also discover that you no longer need to reach for painkillers as frequently, since a significant number of headaches are often caused by an excessive amount of coffee, tea or alcohol.

Taking up some form of physical exercise

If you are sedentary by nature, it is worth considering taking up an enjoyable form of physical exercise that appeals to you. When we take up regular physical activity we can increase overall fitness, improve emotional well-being, boost confidence in improved physical strength and stamina, discourage the development of osteoporosis, and feel more full of energy and vitality than we may have done for years. The most difficult thing when we are feeling low is finding the initial motivation to get going, but once we are over this hurdle and start to enjoy the benefits of regular exercise, we are likely to wonder why on earth it took us so long to get moving. The improvement is due to the increased secretion of chemicals that are natural antidepressants, called endorphins; these are the substances that are responsible for the sense of well-being and euphoria that follows physical exercise. The form of physical activity that is most likely to induce this effect is any form of exercise that gives the heart and lungs a thorough work-out. Possibilities include cycling, running, power walking, or dancing. Once you have discovered a sport or system of exercise that appeals to you, make sure that you are realistic about your goals at the outset so that you don't fall into the trap of being over-ambitious and giving up at the first hurdle. On the other hand, by taking it at a realistic pace at the beginning, you will have the maximum chance of finding that you feel motivated to continue.

Making maximum use of our lung capacity

One of the most impressive benefits of regular aerobic exercise includes an increased ability to breathe more deeply and evenly so that maximum use is made of the oxygen that we breathe in. Because breathing falls into the category of an involuntary function of the body, we may not think too much about the way in which we breathe unless something draws our attention to it, such as feeling unexpectedly breathless or wheezy. On the other hand, many of us tend not to make maximum use of our lung capacity, but tend to breathe in a fairly shallow and rapid way. This tendency is made even more marked and noticeable when we feel stressed, tense or depressed, since our natural reaction to these emotions tends to involve tightening up the muscles of the chest, shoulders and upper arms. As a result of this 'body armouring' we inevitably begin to breathe rapidly, using only a small part of the upper chest, which has the effect of making us feel even more jittery and tense. However, if we learn how to breathe deeply and steadily without getting breathless during aerobic activity, we are supporting our bodies in the vitally important processes of elimination and removal of toxic waste from our systems. The latter are important contributory factors to feeling alert and full of energy: feelings which often suffer greatly when we feel depressed. We can make use of a simple test in order to work out whether we are exercising aerobically. This involves nothing more complicated than seeing if we can maintain a conversation without getting out of breath. If we can do this without strain or signs of breathlessness we are working aerobically. However, if we are gasping for breath, the chances are that we have moved into an anaerobic state which is counter-productive and gives us none of the benefits of working at an aerobic level.

Aromatherapy hints

The following essential oils may be vaporised and inhaled in order to balance erratic moods. Oils include *bergamot, clary sage, coriander* and *ylang ylang*.

Homoeopathic hints

- Mood swings and feeling generally low may respond well to *staphisagria* if there is a general history of suppressed anger. Disproportionate explosive outbursts are likely to be triggered by the most trivial of circumstances as a result of irritation and anger not having being expressed at the right time and to the right person. Mood swings and depression that follow early hysterectomy may be eased considerably by this remedy if other features agree. Symptoms are likely to be made more intense by sexual contact, emotional stress and physical contact. They are eased by being given emotional space, warmth and rest.
- Those who feel tense, 'short-fused', and on an emotional see-saw with regard to mood swings may need *nux vomica*.

Symptoms that respond well to this remedy include classic features of personal and professional burn-out. As well as extremely volatile outbursts of irritability and lack of patience, additional symptoms include stress-related headaches, indigestion, constipation and poor sleep pattern. Those who need *nux vomica* take refuge in stimulants in order to keep up the pace, and alcohol and sleeping tablets to unwind. They are also likely to become physically, emotionally and mentally exhausted by throwing themselves into extra work pressures rather than taking time out to detox and relax.

- Severe mental, emotional and physical exhaustion may do well from treatment with *sepia*. The classic *sepia* state is one of feeling unable to cope with daily domestic and professional demands. Libido is likely to be non-existent, with a general state of indifference to any sexual advances, which are regarded as yet another demand to be satisfied. Moods may swing from irritability to apathy and anxiety, depending on the circumstances. Aerobic exercise in the fresh air is the one thing that helps balance mood swings, and it is wise not to leave long gaps between meals, in order to avoid low blood sugar levels. Symptoms are likely to be more obvious and severe when one is stressed, before a period, and when sitting still and brooding for too long.

- Mood swings with a general sense of feeling bereft and extremely tearful for no obvious reason may be eased considerably by *ignatia*. Although this remedy is most often helpful in situations where bereavement has actually taken place, it's also of great value where a death hasn't occurred, but a relationship may have come to an end. As a result, *ignatia* can be of terrific value when grieving may be taking place for anything from children leaving home, to the break-up of a long-term relationship, or acknowledging the loss of youth. When this remedy is needed, symptoms don't improve with the passing of time, and may seem to actually get more intense and established. *Ignatia* can play a very important part in helping us achieve closure so that we can move on with the rest of our lives.

- Rapid changes of mood that are especially noticeable on waking may do better with *lachesis*. Because of this negative effect of sleep, there may be a real dislike of going to bed, with a tendency to work until the early hours of the morning. Mood swings and depression are closely linked to hormonal fluctuations and as a result, will be especially obvious pre-menstrually or during the menopause. Night sweats are very severe on waking, which adds to a general aversion to, or fear of going to bed. Symptoms are made worse by restrictive clothes around the neck or waist, and stuffy, overheated surroundings. They are relieved by wearing light, loose clothes, cool drinks, and the onset of a period.

- On the other hand, mild depression with very easily provoked weepiness for the most minor reason may be considerably relieved by *pulsatilla*. Along with feeling low there is likely to be a desperate need for sympathy and attention. There is a general sense of huge relief after a good cry on a sympathetic shoulder, and gentle exercise in the fresh air. Symptoms are generally more obvious pre-menstrually and when resting.

Herbal hints

- When feeling emotionally vulnerable or unstable in response to stress and too much pressure, it can be immensely helpful to add a soothing and reviving herbal infusion to your bathwater. Soak three generous handfuls of *lavender* or *lemon balm* in a pan of cold water overnight. The next morning, bring the pan to the boil, strain, and add the infusion to your bathwater as and when it is needed.

- Because of its relaxing effect, *borage* may be taken in infusion form to ease feelings of depression and distress. In addition, because of its reputation for supporting the adrenal glands, it can be especially of value during the menopause when there can be a risk of adrenal exhaustion setting in. *Borage* appears to have the effect of bolstering oestrogen production, thus easing symptoms of hot flushes as well. The infusion may be easily made by adding a cupful of hot water to one teaspoonful of the dried herb, and leaving the infusion to stand for fifteen minutes.

Strain, and then sip as a warm, uplifting drink whenever feeling low or under strain.

- An infusion of any of the following will soothe and uplift the spirits: *camomile* (in order to induce relaxation), *lemon balm* (to ease depression combined with digestive problems), *vervain* (exhausted depression where vitality is very low), or *valerian* (for anxious, agitated depression or mood swings). In order to make an infusion, follow the instructions given above. (**NB!** Avoid *vervain* in pregnancy, and avoid using *valerian* on a routine basis, since prolonged use can give rise to symptoms of palpitations, headaches and muscle spasms.)
- Recent clinical trials have demonstrated that *hypericum* can be extremely effective in easing symptoms of mild to moderate depression. It can be obtained in tincture or tablet form. It has been suggested that this herbal medicine may have an adverse effect when combined with a specific range of prescription drugs, so it is wise to consult your GP or alternative health practitioner if you have any doubts about drug interaction before commencing a course of *hypericum*.
- Diluted tincture of *wild oats* may be taken daily in order to strengthen and support the nervous system. Eight drops of the tincture should be dissolved in a small glass of water and taken each day until energy levels respond. This can be of special value if depression has followed on from a period of severe or protracted stress.

Flower essences

- *Willow* may be very helpful in easing symptoms of depression that are combined with feelings of resentment and bitterness towards others.
- *Star of Bethlehem* may be used to reduce distress and depression that follow on from a severe shock and trauma. The latter may involve anything from witnessing or being involved in an accident, to bereavement or coming to terms with unexpected redundancy or end of a relationship.
- Depression that springs from feelings of inadequacy, guilt or

182

extreme self-criticism may respond positively to *pine*.

- *Mustard* may help bouts of depression, gloom and general despondency that descend out of the blue.
- *Sweet chestnut* may be suitable for episodes of depression and extreme anguish when we may feel we have reached the limits of endurance.
- *Honeysuckle* can help those of us who cling too much to the past and find it very difficult to accept and adapt to change.
- *Wild rose* can give a positive emotional boost when we feel apathetic and resigned to a low, unhappy state.

If more than one flower essence sounds appropriate you can make up a treatment bottle of a combination of essences. For advice on making up a treatment bottle see the 'Flower essences' section of 'Fatigue' on p. 165.

Recommended Reading

Brewer, Sarah, *The Menopause*. Thorsons, 1997.

Campion, Kitty, *Menopause Naturally*. Newleaf, 1998.

Chopra, Deepak, *Ageless Body, Timeless Mind*. Random House, 1993.

Fairley, Josephine and Stacey, Sarah, *Feel Fabulous Forever: The Anti-Ageing Health and Beauty Bible*. Kyle Cathie, 1998.

Fonda, Jane, *Women Coming of Age*. Penguin, 1984.

Glenville, Marilyn, *Natural Alternatives to HRT*. Kyle Cathie, 1997.

Hall, Judy, *Holistic Menopause: A New Approach to Midlife Change*. Findhorn Press, 1998.

Howell, Donna, *The Unofficial Guide to Coping with Menopause*. Macmillan USA, 1999.

Hunniford, Gloria and De Vries, Jan, *Feel Fabulous Over Fifty*. Hodder and Stoughton, 2000.

Ikenzie, Ifeoma, *Menopause and Homoeopathy: A Guide to Women in Midlife*. North Atlantic Books, 1998.

Kenton, Leslie, *Passage to Power: Natural Menopause Revolution*. Random House, 1995.

Kenton, Leslie, *Ten Steps to a Younger You*. Vermilion, 2000.

Lalvani, Vimla, *Stop the Age Clock*. Hamlyn, 1998.

Lee, John, *What Your Doctors May Not Tell You about Perimenopause: Balance Your Hormones and Your Life from Thirty to Fifty.* Warner Books, 1999.

MacEoin, Beth, *Homoeopathy and the Menopause: A Natural and Effective Way to Manage Your Change of Life.* Thorsons, 1996.

MacEoin, Beth, *Natural Medicine: A Practical Guide to Family Health.* Bloomsbury, 1999.

MacEoin, Beth, *Come Alive: Your Six Point Plan for Lasting Health and Energy.* Hodder and Stoughton, 2000.

McIntyre, Anne, *The Complete Woman's Herbal: A Manual of Healing Herbs and Nutrition for Personal Well-Being and Family Care.* Gaia, 1994.

Northrup, Christine, *Women's Bodies, Women's Wisdom: The Complete Guide to Women's Health and Well-Being.* Piatkus, 1998.

Phillips, Angela and Rakusen, Jill, *The New Our Bodies, Ourselves.* Penguin, 1989.

Spillane, Mary and McKee, Victoria, *Ultrahealth: Everywoman's Guide to Facing the Future.* Macmillan, 1999.

Stoppard, Miriam, *Natural Menopause.* Dorling Kindersley, 1998.

Vyas, Bharti, *Simply Radiant: Practical Techniques to Turn Back the Years.* Thorsons, 1999.

Wildwood, Chrissie, *The Bloomsbury Encyclopedia of Aromatherapy.* Bloomsbury, 1996.

Wilson, Robert, *Understanding HRT and the Menopause: Managing 'The Change' with or without Hormone Replacement Therapy.* Penguin, 1992.

Useful Addresses

National

UK

British Acupuncture Council
Park House
206–208 Latimer Road
London
W10 6RE

Telephone: 020 8964 0222

Society of Teachers of the Alexander Technique
20 London House
266 Fulham Road
London
SW10 9EL

Telephone: 020 7351 0828

Aromatherapy Organisations Council
PO Box 355
Croydon
CR9 2QP

Telephone: 020 8251 7912

British Association for Autogenic Training and Therapy
Royal London Homoeopathic Hospital
Great Ormond Street
London
WC1N 3HR

Telephone: 020 7837 8833

Chinese Herbal Medicine
Register of Chinese Herbal Medicine
PO Box 400
Wembley
Middlesex
HA9 9NZ

Telephone: 020 7224 0883

British Complementary Medical Association
249 Fosse Road
Leicester
LE3 1AE

Telephone: 0116 282 5511

Council for Complementary and Alternative Medicine
Park House
206–208 Latimer Road
London
W10 6RE

Telephone: 020 8968 3862

The Society of Homoeopaths
4a Artizan Road
Northampton
NN1 4HU

Telephone: 01604 621400

National Institute of Medical Herbalists
56 Longbrook Street
Exeter
EX4 6AH

Telephone: 01392 426022

Natural Progesterone Information Service
BCM BOX 4315
London
WC1N 3XX

The Nutri Centre
7 Park Crescent
London
W1N 3HE

Telephone: 020 7436 5122

British Association of Nutritional Therapists
PO Box 2656
Lewes
East Sussex
BN8 6QN

Telephone: 01825 872 921

National Osteoporosis Society
PO Box 10
Radstock
Bath
BA3 3UB

Telephone: 01761 432472

The British Wheel of Yoga
1 Hamilton Place
Boston Road
Sleaford
Lincolnshire
NG34 7ES

Telephone: 01529 306851

International

Australia

Association of Traditional Health Practitioners Incorporated
PO Box 346
Elizabeth, South Australia 5112

Telephone: 08 8284 2324

Canada

Acupuncture Canada
107 Leitch Drive
Grimsby, Ontario
L3M 2T9

Telephone: 905 563 8930

The Canadian Herb Society
5251 Oak Street
Vancouver, BC
V6M 4H1

Tzu Chi Institute for Complementary Medicine
715 West 12th Avenue
Health Centre
4th Floor West
Vancouver, BC
V5Z 1M9

Telephone: 604 875 4769

USA

American Association of Acupuncture and Oriental Medicine
4101 Lake Boone Trail
Suite 201
Raleigh, NC 27607

Telephone: 919 787 5181

American Aromatherapy Association
PO Box 3679
South Passadena, CA 91031

Telephone: 818 457 1742

American Chiropractic Association
1701 Clarendon Blvd
Arlington, VA 22209

Telephone: 703 276 8800

American Herbalist Guild
PO Box 1683
Soquel, CA 95073

National Center for Homoeopathy
801 North Fairfax Street
Suite 306
Alexandria, VA 22314

Telephone: 703 548 7790

International Association of Yoga Therapists
109 Hillside Avenue
Mill Valley, CA 94941

Telephone: 415 383 4587

Index

adrenal glands 42, 66, 99–100
adrenaline 43, 66, 100, 149
aerobic exercise 57, 100–1, 179,
   180
age, at menopause 22–3
ageing 11–12, 37–40
alcohol 70–2, 73, 120, 123,
   153–4, 177
Alexander Technique 106,
   112–14
alternative therapies 12–14,
   15–17, 24
   and HRT 125–7, 130–4
   self-help for short-term
     symptoms 137–83
androgens 26, 42
anti-oxidant nutrients 77–9, 84,
   89, 90, 91

anxiety 55, 72, 103, 139, 141,
   144
   diet and 148–9
   exercise and 149–50
   herbal and homoeopathic
     remedies 150–2
   symptoms 145, 150–1
aqua aerobics 105
aromatherapy 140, 143, 150,
   154, 162, 171, 179
autogenic training 57–8

balance 14–16, 35, 36–7, 52
   see also hormone balance
beta-carotene 77–8, 89
blood sugar levels 65–7, 71,
   140, 158, 159, 160
body maintenance 93–5

body sculpting 106, 108
bone density 23, 71, 90, 120–1, 133
    exercise and 94, 98–100, 107, 109
    see also osteoporosis
boron 90
breathing techniques 55–6, 110–11, 146–7, 161–2, 178–9

caffeine 67, 72, 120, 160, 176–7
calcium 68, 80–1, 89
    dietary sources 81–2, 88
cancers 75, 76, 125
change, responses to 5–6, 36, 38
cholesterol 83–4
Chopra, Deepak 40
circulatory disease 71, 72
climateric 21
coffee *see* caffeine
cognitive therapy 49
complex carbohydrates 66, 159, 160
constipation 69
contraception, freedom from 29
co-ordination 109, 111
cosmetic surgery 35, 36
curiosity 38
cycling 105

dairy foods 68
dancing 105
degenerative disease 89
delegation 54
depression 12, 171, 173–7

alternative self-help 179–83
    diet and 175–7
    exercise and 102–3, 177–8
diet 62, 63–9
    anxiety and 148–9
    depression and 175–7
    energy and 158–61
    fluid retention and 166–7
    heart disease and 122
    hot flushes and 139, 140
    libido and 170
    osteoporosis and 64, 68, 69, 71, 72, 79–82, 119–20
    sleep and 154
dietary supplements 86–91

eating disorders 23
EFAs (essential fatty acids) 73–4, 75–6
emotional well-being 98
    exercise and 102–3, 112–13
energy 94, 97, 156–7
    diet and 158–61
exercise 85, 103–14, 177–8
    aerobic 57, 100–1, 179, 180
    anxiety and 149–50
    balanced approach 94–5
    benefits 92–3, 96–103, 139–40
    osteoporosis and 98, 120
expectations of menopause 20, 23–4, 33

fat 68, 73–9, 84, 85, 159
fatigue 55, 72, 87, 129, 156–8
    diet and 158–61

herbal and homoeopathic
    remedies 162–5
fibre 68–9
flexibility 38
    muscular 108, 110, 111, 112
flower essences 152, 165,
    182–3
fluid retention 165–8
food cravings 97

GPs, conventional approach to
    menopause 18, 63, 126, 131,
    134–5

health 9–10, 28, 35
    impact of stress on 41–2
heart disease 134
    diet and 64, 75, 76, 82–6
    exercise and 97, 100–2, 107,
        122
    HRT and 117, 122
    risk factors 122
    smoking and 71
herbal medicines
    for anxiety 151–2
    for fatigue 164
    for fluid retention 168
    for hot flushes 141–2
    for loss of libido 172–3
    for mood swings 181–2
    for night sweats 144
    for sleep disturbance 156
homoeopathic medicines 13
    for anxiety 150–1
    for fatigue 163–4
    for fluid retention 167–8

for hot flushes 140–1
for loss of libido 171–2
for mood swings 179–81
for night sweats 143
for sleep disturbance 154–5
hormone balance 73–4, 99,
    128–9
    see also HRT (hormone
        replacement therapy)
hot flushes 55, 72, 98, 117,
    138–40
    herbal and homoeopathic
        remedies 140–2
HRT (hormone replacement
    therapy) 18–19, 29, 63–4,
    134–6
    contraindications 124–5
    early days 10–12
    heart and 82–3
    osteoporosis and 117, 120–1
    side effects 124
    types of 124–5

immune system 75, 89, 91, 99

jogging 98, 107, 120
junk food 65, 158, 176

Lee, John 127, 129
libido, loss of 168–73
life expectancy 97

magnesium 91
meditation 58–9, 147–8
metabolic rate 97
mind 32, 34, 41

mood swings 47, 173–9
  herbal and homoeopathic
    remedies 179–83
motherhood 28, 173
muscle strength 94, 95, 99, 108,
  109, 111

night sweats 55, 142–3
  herbal and homoeopathic
    remedies 143–4
nutrition see 62, 63–9

oestrogen 15, 26, 42, 76, 116
oestrogen dominance 68, 74,
  127–30
organisation 52–3
osteoporosis 118
  diet and 64, 68, 69, 71, 72,
    79–82, 119–20
  exercise and 98, 120
  HRT and 117, 120–1
  natural progesterone and
    129–30
  risk factors 119, 133
  smoking and 83
Our Bodies, Ourselves 9–10
ovaries 21, 23

panic attacks 144–52
periods
  changes in pattern 22, 25
  freedom from 29
personal relationships 46–7
physical fitness 32–3
  see also exercise
phytoestrogens 76

Pilates 106, 110–11
positivity 19–20, 29–31, 40
posture 111, 112, 113
pre-menopause 21–2
premature menopause 22–3
preparation for menopause
  34–61
prioritisation of tasks 51–2
professional role 39
progesterone cream 126–8,
  129–30
puberty 7–8, 24–7

racket games 98, 107
red meat 67–8, 143
relatives, experience of
  menopause 19
relaxation 50, 54–5, 139, 151,
  154, 161
  background to 55–7
  techniques 57–61
retirement 30

salt 69–70
selenium 91
self-esteem 27, 36, 48–9, 102
sex life 29–30
  see also libido, loss of
Simonton, C. and S.M. 41
skin-brushing techniques
  162
skin condition 71, 90, 127
sleep patterns 72, 88, 152–4,
  158
  diet and 148, 154
  stress and 55, 56–7

herbal and homoeopathic remedies for disturbance 154–6
smoking 19–20, 71, 83, 120, 123
social life 38–9, 175
soya products 76–7, 85
stamina 94, 95, 109
stimulants 65, 67, 72
stress 42–3, 45, 171
  impact on health 41–2
  negative 39–40, 41, 42–3
  personal 44, 46–9
  work-related 44
stress reduction 44
  exercise and 99, 100, 108
  personal stress 46–9
  relaxation and 54–61
  work-related 49–54
sugar 66–7
  see also blood sugar levels

swimming 105
symptoms 21–2, 27, 116–17
  alternative therapies and 16–17, 137–83
  HRT and 11–12, 117
  see also under individual symptoms

T'ai chi 106, 111–12
time management 49–50

vitamins 78, 81, 89–90, 149

walking 99, 105, 120
weight 20, 116
weight training 106
workload, evaluating 53–4

xenoestrogens 127–8

yoga 99, 106, 108–10